The secret healer has got

stress in her sights

and she's about to

make a killing.

To my lovely dad....

You used to tell me "*Get it done*"

So I did.

This is book is for you.

Let me ask you, where are *you* in your career at the moment? Newly qualified or flying high with the stars? What are you looking to get out of your vocation? What do you want to achieve?

Instinct tells me the fact you have chosen this book (thanks for that by the way!) means your sales figures are not looking as good as they should be. Even if they are, a really great business person is always looking for their sales to go up and up. The problem is...who on earth really *wants* to sell?

Let's face it **sell** is a four letter word. It is rude and crude and dare I say it, certainly not very British. Your problem is this:

Sales is the only thing in your business which increases profit.

Everything else is a cost.

Love it or hate it, the reality is if you have chosen to build a business, it's no good sitting about twiddling your thumbs. Customers don't turn up uninvited, let's be honest, frankly that's rude. They won't pry into your business and ask you how much you charge, because it simply isn't done. They might gossip behind your back to find out what you're up to but they certainly won't ask you to your face. The problem is if you want someone to become your customer...***you really do have to tell them***.

Here's the thing. I am English. I live in a genteel town. I understand polite. But I'm telling you, people, whilst there certainly is etiquette to sales, waiting to be asked plays absolutely no part.

You simply have to seek out conversations.

Read that again.

I didn't say soliloquies, pitches, or aggressive sales force. All success is going to take is a few well chosen words, asked at the right time and with the right words in reply. Oh and the gumption to get off your **** and stop wishing for profit and the wherewithal to get out there and find it.

I can even tell you where those sales are. In fact in this book, I do. Backed up with clinical reports, statistics and some medical terminology to boot, you can knock on doors with literally hundreds of pounds of spending power behind them and realistically expect them to open.

Do you want to know what to say? Here are the scripts, the tools and techniques to get you the sale. Then the next one, the next and the next!

Worried about what to charge? Yep I was too, that's why I have broken down stats and figures to tell you how much people will pay, for what, and for how long.

The problem is of course, by nature as healers we are *not* salesmen. We like a softly, softly approach and we certainly don't want to be seen as pushy, so we back off from sales. Our businesses fall behind and the dream we had of making people better fades behind other part time jobs we have to take, or worse still, red letter bills.

If your business is floundering, not only can I tell you why, but I can give you the tools to fix it. In *The Professional Stress Solution* I filled in the healing blanks to put your therapy on the fierce clinical footing to outstrip not only many of the aromatherapists in your country, but the entire world over. In **this** book I teach you the marketing knowhow to reach those target clients and to close your deals.

Aromatherapy courses are wonderful. I loved every second of mine. You spend hours thinking about glorious scents, you write essays about digestion, reproduction and the extraction of oil, but when it comes to the nitty gritty of getting your business up and running, the lessons are scarce on the ground. You may understand the insurance connotations and how to design your leaflets, but how many of you have actually learned how to sell?

I don't mean the stuff a double-glazing salesman does or even the cosmetics women in Boots. I am talking about soft consultative sell where you ask the patient what they want and then you deliver exactly what they feel they need. I know you can sell, because I can! It's as simple as that.

It took me 20 years to amass the sales experience I needed, the underpinning knowledge of other therapies and a very watchful eye to see how the healing market has changed. On the surface it may seem like the aromatherapy market is saturated, but trust me it is about to explode. Aromatherapy is no longer fringe science. It has clinical trials backing it up, funding in hospitals, and when hospices and special schools run out of ideas, they turn to us.

And when the market does go boom....I want to make sure talented aromatherapists have the wherewithal to sail the tsunami it will create.

Here's how I'm going to do that...

I have spent years perfecting phraseology and pitch. I want to give that expertise to you. I have read thousands of manuals and made literally millions of calls. Some were good, some were bad and some secured me six figure contracts. I can show you how.

This is what I offer....

- Strategic indicators of where to find your business

- Statistical data to help you support your claims

- Clear, in depth sales training and scripts to help you construct your calls

- The marketing strategies to improve your business 10 fold *at least*

- Best of all you will see your business achieve the potential you always knew it could, but sadly have been watching in frustration and bewilderment as somehow it just *wouldn't.*

- See that arrow on the front cover? When you launch it, it will land right smack on target...I promise.

Table of contents

Chapter 1 Who is this know it all woman anyway?

Fair question and I'll try to answer it fully because I want you to be reassured I have things which are useful for you to hear.

I qualified as an aromatherapist in 1993. I was born into the aromatherapy family business, and was trained by my mother and step father. I still consider these people to be two of the best healers I have ever met. On my Anatomy and Physiology paper I got 100% and 98% on my aromatherapy paper (Cade took two marks away from me and I was so annoyed I have never used the oil again). I joined the IFA and completed the Advanced Diploma of Aromatherapy with honours.

The healing world was at my feet, right?

Wrong.

Like many of you, I was so excited I had passed my diploma I stood there and rubbed my hands in glee. What is it they said in Field of Dreams? "If you build it they will come?" Well I did build it in terms of qualifications and knowledge, but after the case histories were completed, nobody came!

I write this in May 2014. Actually in August it will be 21 years since I sat my exams. The world looks very different geographically. There is no longer a Czechoslovakia. Hong Kong now belongs to China and there are now many different Baltic States. Who could have guessed the princess who occupied every news front page would sadly now be dead and the US would have black president? In 1993, I had never even used the internet, let alone considered writing books for Amazon!

In that time the face of aromatherapy has changed unrecognisably too.

I was already working in an aromatherapy firm in '93. Jill Bruce Aromatherapy, (later to become The Apothecary) travelled to craft and agricultural shows selling their wares. I administered the training school and wrote their newsletter. Back then if I showed customers an essential oil preparation to help their headache, they looked at me in disbelief. The idea of swallowing a pill made far more sense than rubbing something into their heads.

In many ways the growth of aromatherapy has been its own downfall. As the fireworks went off to herald the Millennium, lavender and tea tree were on every supermarket shelf. People learned that oils were relaxing and invigorating and the cosmetics industry went wild for their gorgeous scents. Magazines regaled how sniffing a bottle of oil would relax you and help you to get to sleep, but information stopped there. Now everyone from my postman to Goldie Hawn will recommend some essential oils to calm, but how many people know they are capable of so much more?

There is very little information in *The Secret Healer* books which the Jill Bruce School of Aromatherapy did not teach back in '93, in fact a great deal of the therapy books come straight from my Advanced Aromatherapy lesson notes. The thing is though the public's perception of our skill has changed. They know what aromatherapy is now...especially in terms of stress. The problem is therapists are still not equipped to deal with either the public's or the doctors' new found acceptances of it.

In '99, I became suffocated working and living with family so decided to make a break. Almost by accident I fell into a role of recruitment consultant, which I don't mind telling you wasn't even what I thought it was! I'd imagined it to be a lovely altruistic role finding people new jobs. The truth of a career which was 80% telesales cold calling came as something of a rather rude shock.

After the first week on the phones I was ready to take out a hit on receptionists and I absolutely hated my new career, then at 4 o'clock on Friday I picked up my first job. The voice on the end of the phone said "I need a receptionist for Monday", to which I replied "OK, thanks", and immediately replaced the receiver in panic! Much to mine and my manager's relief my selling prowess very quickly began to improve. Within 12 months I was the most successful permanent recruitment consultant in the company. Then my phone began to ring and headhunters were queuing up at the door.

I loved my job but by 2008 I'd had enough. I wanted out of the rat race and then the universe decided she had had enough too. After years of gently nudging, she decided to give me a great big kick in the guts. First I discovered I was pregnant (in a scan to see if I needed a hysterectomy!), and then I suffered a massive blood clot in my lung. Although not anywhere as dramatic as you see on TV, it does poleaxe you into bed. I couldn't breathe, let alone talk on the phone, so I had to find a new way to sell.

After building a couple of websites, I looked for people who might *pay* me to write. There I discovered ghost writing, the world's coolest and weirdest job! I found out people would give me money just to write about stuff I loved. My first job was a recipe book of cheesecakes and a rather strange phenomenon grew from there. Today (end June 14) I rank as number 49 in a pool of a quarter of a million writers. I have written 7 books which have gone to number one in their genre on Amazon, most of them about natural healing. I suspect I may be the most published aromatherapy writer you have never heard of! So, as well as selling, I also know a lot about the internet, in particular e-books.

Right now I suspect the internet, marketing's greatest ally, could potentially be aromatherapy's most dangerous threat. Much of the information on the web is rehashed rubbish featuring the same old information. Many of Amazon's books are written by people who have never even picked up a bottle of oil. Consequently although I can give you real evidence of people wanting to know more about what you do, most of the time they go away feeling, frankly, despondent about what they read. Sadly they seek other therapies to sort out their problems, and your potential client database is lost.

Well, I for one intend to make some changes. This is me, stepping up to be counted for a start. Right here, right now, I want you to think about how *you* can shout louder and clearer to drown out this marketing hype. Let's see what you can do to set the record straight.

People, it's time to man up!

For the main part aromatherapy is a feminine art. Whilst there are some truly extraordinary male therapists, Robert Tisserand, Gabriel Mojay and Daniel Penoel to name just a few, statistically the volume of women on the practitioners' register far outstrips the number of men.

Herein lays a potential difficulty for essential oil based healing. Our greatest attribute, our gentle, feminine, healing natures can often stand in the way of our own success. For the rulers of the sales world are men. More saliently the marketing gurus of the internet are men. So those who are making a killing, and raking in the revenue from our oils and essential oil information, are potentially not healers at all.

So, ladies and gentlemen, forget the lavender oil, it's time to wake up and smell the coffee. You simply have to start selling. Don't let that worry you. In *Sales Strategies for Gentle Souls* I'll show you where your customers are, how to target them and even how to maximise your profit margin in the process. It's easy (hard work potentially, but certainly not difficult) and as a woman I can tell you really good quality selling is really fun when you know how.

Chapter 2 Do you know where your target is?

Those of you who have read *The Professional Stress Solution* have the tools and techniques to smash your competition out of the water, but there are five questions you need to ask yourself.

- Who are your customers?

- Do you know how to bump into them?

- What will you say when you meet them?

- Who is your competition?

- How can you beat them?

Hopefully already you kind of know, but let's break it down.

Identifying target markets

The newspapers tell us one in three of us suffers from stress. I am not sure if that is true, I suppose it maybe so, but *I* couldn't find any evidence that really backed that up. So I wanted to find out more. Here's what I found.

Globally **110 million people a year** die from the effects of stress. That accounts for 7 people every 2 seconds.

I know! It made me feel sick!

What's more, putting my analytical brain on for a moment, that figure pertains to the global total. I wouldn't have thought people in the Sudan or Papua New Guinea or Easter Island or wherever would have a significant number of their deaths attributed to the term *stress*. Maybe, I don't know, it's a predominately Western world epidemic so the stats are potentially skewed. In fact then, of that 110 million, a large percentage are likely to be eg. American, Australian and European.

So then I wanted to look specifically at Britain's problem for the sake of my own business. If you are working in a different country, the process is simple and the same.

I started with looking at the health service statistics. The NHS turned to RoSPA for their evidence. For those of you unclear this is the Royal Society for the Prevention of Accidents. It seems a fairly good place for them to start.

Work Related Stress

Their statistics tell us that 400,000 workers are operating under high levels of work related stress.

The Health and Safety Executive report that in 2011/2012 out of 1,073,000 work related absences a massive 428,000 were attributed to stress. That is 40%.

But when I read further I found a report by the mental health charity MIND from 2010 which states that one in five people (19%) say yes, they have called in to work sick but 93% of them admitted to lying to their bosses about the reason why. If that is true then the figure is *significantly* higher.

The HSE have made very detailed reports about where these stressed souls are most likely to be Sadly, there are no surprises here.

Highest at risk over a three-year period were health professionals, and in particular nurses. (See the effects of shift work on the body in *The Professional Stress Solution*). Next on the list came our teachers and education staff. The caring and welfare staff followed closely behind, including housing workers.

I suppose that we are not likely to see your one-man bands and small businesses in these findings because a) their occupations are too diverse to make it into the figures and b) they do not have the official reporting structures of the big boys. Nevertheless this is useful data.

CIPD (these are the people who are in charge of personnel officers) say that estimated costs to UK business amount to £13 billion p.a. In the public sector the average employee sickness level is 9.1 days at a cost of £800 per employee. In the private sector it is less, 6.4 days at a cost of £476 per employee.

Now that ladies and gentleman is a hell of a figure.

For a second let's recap on what we have found out there.

- The problem of stress is not just an issue about not being able to relax, it is having very real effects on industry and our economy.

- There are literally hundreds of millions of potential patients who need to get fixed.

- We know where most of the problem areas are .

- Lastly, we now know how much we can charge.

How many of you thought *"Do we?"* ?

We do. Because anything under £476 is saving a company money, and will bring you far more customers than looking for just one patient. Canvass the company and you have loads of potential sales.

So we know then that stress patients can be found at work. What else?

Marital Stress

A recent article in the Telegraph told an interesting tale of a study undertaken by one Nancy Levy for the University of Utah. She speaks of how her group had suspected that being in a stressful relationship may lead a person to have increased levels of blood pressure, obesity and cholesterol, which in turn may relate to metabolic syndrome, one of the main problems behind heart disease and diabetes.

The findings were fascinating, and when I read it I had to sit for a good while and ponder why.

They found that yes, they could make a direct link between relationship stress and heart disease....but only in women. Men did not process the stress in the same physiological way.

I'm still pondering. I don't know why but there are lots of issues about heart chakras, pituitary glands and *Men are from Mars* swimming round. Certainly the responses we found in *The*

Professional Stress Solution about the way women process stress on the opposite amygdala to men may hold some clues.

What is important though is the middle step. Metabolic syndrome...they are getting fat. So these people are found at slimming groups, gyms, relationship support meetings and relaxation groups....or maybe they are just wandering round wearing leggings they shouldn't! That might be another clue.

Stress related disease

In 2010 I was asked to work on a voluntary basis with a proposed organisation called the Walsall Independent Treatment Centre. It would provide the long awaited gateway, the rainbow bridge if you will, between the allopathic and complementary worlds of medicine.

Its structure and viability hung on a white paper that the, then newly incumbent, Health Secretary Andrew Lansley had published. It detailed the proposal of a reform of the NHS where GPs would take control of commissioning care for their patients' needs based on their requirements and desires at that time. It worked on the fundamental principle that each person in the country would have their own pot of money to spend on their care as they wished. Control would be passed from the primary care trusts and placed squarely at the feet of the GPs.

Some of this you will know because what ensued was media frenzy about the uproar and dissent within the ranks. GPs were enraged about the role they were being asked to play, and had no experience or training to do. Eventually, after their success in lobbying every resource available to them, Lansley was forced to review the reform strategy.

My job was to consult on the complementary medicine side of things alongside a group of 9 doctors based in the UK and the States. The job of writing the promotional material fell to me. Sadly the centre never came to fruition because of the massive size of the project for outreached funding potential and also the veto of the reform. Nevertheless the principles I discovered remain firm.

At first, selling complementary services to GPs seemed impossible to me. But actually when researched, with both GPs and commissioning units, it became clear that not only were they completely open to the idea, they very much wanted it. One particular unit held control of every one of 250 GP surgeries in the Worcestershire area and wanted to roll out the business model in all of them.

The key lies in 2 very specific areas, which GPs find nebulous and a waste of their time and resources - they are just waiting for an opportunity to present itself that means that they can offload them. These areas are **advocacy** and **somatisation.** I'll explain these more in a moment.

Far from being a closed door to complementary therapies, the average GP is now quite enlightened as to what can be offered and agrees that emotional and spiritual distress does indeed underlie a large proportion of the presenting illnesses they see. Further, they see the patient's self care, for things like COPD for instance, as fundamental to keeping their care costs to a minimum. Preventative medicine reducing the number of their repeat visits is seen as the most effective method of helping them to achieve their own profitability objectives.

So how can you get your hands on that business?

Advocacy is someone else's job unless you *particularly* want to do it. It is representing people in court or hospital meetings and generally fighting the corner of the underdog. Over simplified but you catch my drift.

Somatisation, though, that could very soon become your favourite word.

It is a psychiatric term and its dictionary definition is

the manifestation of psychological distress by the presentation of bodily symptoms.

Feel enlightened? No, of course you don't because aromatherapists have known this happens for *like forever, man*!

We are talking about two differing levels here.

Somatisation might manifest in symptoms such as

- Chest pains

- Tiredness

- Dizziness

- Back pain

- Feeling sick (nauseated)

Those worst affected are deemed to have **somatoform disorders.**

These are more specific physical manifestations with unexplainable roots. Potentially there can be many tests and procedures done, none of which provide any answers except "Just put it down to stress". They can be closely, but not precisely, aligned to psychosomatic disorders. Similar, probably related, but not necessarily the same.

These may present as

- Somatisation disorder
- Hypochondria
- Conversion disorder
- Body dysmorphic disorder
- Pain disorder

In fact, statistics show that in 2008/9 Primary Care Trusts in England spent a massive £3 billion on treating these Medically Unexplained Symptoms (MUS) which was.....wait for it...

10% of the NHS budget for the work force age population! This was made up of prescription charges, test costs and appointment consultation times.

No wonder they want rid of it!

That's OK. We'll have it!

And of course it goes without saying this stress epidemic has the same effects throughout the western world. Whilst these stats pertain to Britain, the potential opportunities are worldwide.

Pick up the phone to the practice manager or make an appointment to see the partners. They will explain to you whether they need you to get registered with the commissioning unit or they can do direct referrals.

Look out for expert patient days and also the patient support meetings, to get your face seen by patients who might be looking for help. Make sure your business card says you treat stress *and related disorders*.

From a patient's point of view, benefits abound when they can spend time with a holistic practitioner and not just have to fit their woes into a fifteen minute slot. That is no criticism of GPs, they have a large number of people to see in a very short time. For many people that works, for others maybe not.

Ok we know where that target market is, but the hard thing is knowing what to say.

I promised you sales conversations, and sales conversations you will have. In this chapter though, let's just think a little about mindset.

The only thing that contributes to profit is sales.

Everything else in your business is a cost.

Uh-oh! That's a scary thought isn't it? Yup, but that's the truth of any business, most pertinently of yours.

The only way you will make more money is if you see more people.

Advertising...costs

Marketing....costs

Using your essential oils.....*mega* costs!

Ask yourself now, does 'sell' still feel like a four letter word?

Here's the thing - I am a good sales person and I have some really good skills, but I only got them through practice. I do have a secret weapon that makes me far better than most. I can outsell most people on the planet, not because I have inherited the gift of the gab, or because I have the strongest close.

I sell so well, because I sell! Most people just don't. They are scared to pick up the phone, they don't feel comfortable speaking to people at their stall and they don't say to customers "why don't you come?"

I promise you, that is the only difference. But why does this happen?

There are two reasons: fear and lack of incentive.

Let's talk about the latter first.

Imagine you worked for me doing telesales and I said to you "sell me a pot of cream for £15, when you do I'll give you £2 commission".

You'd be excited for a bit, but not for very long. All the "No"s would soon grind you down. How many might you sell in a week? Three, maybe four?

What about then if I said to you Gordon at the next desk is still spending his last bonus cheque. I'll do the same for you. Sell 50 in a month and I'll give you £1000 on top of your £2 a pot.

OOO, the call numbers just went up, didn't they?(Lazy so and sos, fancy me having to dangle a carrot like that!) Firstly you want the extra cash, but also you now know it is possible because Gordon's done it, so perhaps you are a bit rubbish and had better sort yourself out!

Here's a quick analogy about what you believe to be possible.

There was once a rock climber in the Alps and he performed amazing, daring feats of height. He scaled faces no-one else could dream of and he had set his sights on this certain one.

For weeks tourists flocked to see him try to conquer this particular face but he could never quite stretch his foot to the next ledge or get his fingers to find the right hole. His deadline of 40 days loomed close and on day 39 he declared it impossible to do. He felt utterly defeated, but resolved his fight was over. His next day's try would be his last.

His climbing companions were exasperated. They had seen him scale far bigger rocks before. They had to find a way to get him to the top. Together, they hatched a plan.

Next morning, the climber looked in horror and dismay to see chalk marks leading to the top. Someone else had broken the face. He had been beaten to the top! Furious, he followed the marks and very easily and with very little effort he reached its precious summit. Bewildered, he couldn't quite work out why everyone was jubilantly laughing when he felt all was lost. Then he saw the rope.

The rope was tied to a tree at the top and had been used to guide his friends *down*. Carefully they had shown him which crags would get him to the top and had marked them in chalk. No-one had beaten him at all. Because he believed the climb was possible, he easily reached the top.

The Secret Healer and her stag

On the front of my books is a thinner version of a lady who looks a bit like me and with her is often her stag. The beautiful, gentle creature is the symbol of the fertility and healing god Cernunnos. He embodies everything I love about the healing arts - quiet, subtle and really so majestic in their effects. The reason I picked him is because the ancients would watch the deer to see which herbs they chose to eat. Their choices were the most succulent and most effective for healing. The deer however is skittish. Whilst it will enter into a ruck with one of its own, it knows its place at the bottom of the food chain. It likes to hide away on its own.

Here, let's go back for a minute to what I said about reasons for not trying to sell. Fear will really do you down. No-one wants to look stupid or have to suffer the effects of someone saying "no". Let me tell you at this point you need to learn a skill set.

When someone says to you "no" in a sales context, seven out of eight times what they mean is "no, not yet"....

So persistence, practice and perspicacity need to become your watch words or you can take on my way into the third, fourth and fifth calls to a prospect, and introduce yourself as their friendly stalker.

You can convert prospects. You will convert prospects. You just have to believe...

By all means be the stag...in your treatment room, but you have to get out there in the sunshine and start hunting too.

Hunt or be hunted.

Darwin got it right....survival of the fittest.

We'll go into the training now but I want you to keep in mind how this can work for you. How you can alter and mould it, because Chapter 5 is important. To thine own self be true. I don't want you to change. I want to help you develop.

So now let's start working out.

Chapter 3 Prospecting

The first thing I need to do is offer you an apology. If you have ever had irritating telesales calls selling catalogue subscriptions or cheaper phone deals during Coronation Street or serving up tea, I potentially had a part to play in that and I am, truly and deeply, sorry. Potentially I may go to hell for the horror I inflicted on this country. Hopefully this book will make amends.

I have, in my time, recruited hundreds of telesales people and trained a fair few too.

Business to consumer calls are hard (because no-one really wants to hear about cheaper landlines). Business to business, well, that's a good deal easier if you know some tricks of the trade. Whilst the tips in the book are telesales skills they will improve every aspect of your selling, and you might find you run your life a little differently too. From this second on I want you to think of these as your life skills. After all they will come to be how you make your living.

A couple of abbreviations to help us on our way, two are real, one is made up -

B2B – Business to business – you are calling a company to sell your business.

B2C – Business to consumer – you are calling to interrupt mum serving up tea.

B2D – Business to doctor – totally made up but it kinda works!

Spotting new business opportunities

Get in the habit of always looking for new business. I am sure you think you already do, but I would suggest you don't. Look at every big company as a potential time bomb waiting to go off. Look for speaking opportunities where you can get your message across. Seek out opportunities to bump into the people with frowns on their face.

Then when you see them, don't freeze!

I have a current gripe. Why do people with amazing skills and talents dumb them down? Are you doing that or do you knowledgably (and engagingly) tell people what you can do?

Let's break down the ways to tell people what you do first.

Feature Advantage Benefit

Let me ask you - Why do *you* buy something? My initial response might be because it's cheap. But actually if I didn't want it, that wouldn't make me buy. Is it because I want it then? Well yes, but why do I want it? The reason why I buy something is because it benefits me in some way.

I buy Tesco big pants because they are comfortable. I buy magic pants because they hide my baby (and cakes) belly and make me look svelte. I buy books because they help me to improve my business, and I buy new frying pans because I can't bear to use the one I have scratched the non-stick off any longer.

It doesn't matter what your product, you can always get someone to buy from you if you offer them the right benefit at the right price.

So conversely, to prove my point:

Last week I saw some Jimmy Choos in the charity shop for £13. They were too small for me, so I didn't buy. The benefit of wearing was not there so my brain didn't really click in. Later I realised I had missed a different benefit...if I put them on eBay, I could make a killing! Now that benefit *did* push me to buy. So back to town I traipsed. Sadly some other lucky gal saw *her* benefit first and is a whole pair of delicious shoes richer.

If we analyse it more, the fault was not entirely my own. The shop had failed to sell the shoes effectively. They had told me the ***features*** of their product but had not pointed out the benefits.

Let me show you.

Jimmy Choo Silver Shoes

6 inch heel

Diamantée detailing

Excellent condition

£12.99

I know, I know! They sound gorgeous and they were and I am an idiot! I know!

Let's just move on.

What would be the ***advantages*** of buying these shoes?

- They would go with loads of clothes

- I would be a lot taller

- They would shape my calves

- They would add a bit of bling

- They would be a great name to add my wardrobe

But what about the benefits of the Jimmy Choos?

The benefits are:

They would go with lots of clothes: they make good financial sense, I get to show off my bling with a million other outfits, I am going to get seen by loads of people in my fabulous shoes

I would be taller: massive benefit for the woman they call Gimli Son of Gloin, I need every inch I can get. There is also a lot to be said for the wisdom on the T Shirt that said I am not fat I am under tall; taller....slimmer looking. I get to look down on someone else for a change. I would look like I had more authority. I could reach everything I wanted in the supermarket. I'd get that catwalk strut models get when they don their heels. My posture would look ace!

They would shape my calves: Ladies, my legs may be short fat and hairy, but they look fantastic! However everyone needs a bit of help.

They would add a bit of bling: Glamour, sass, elegance and sparkle. Who doesn't need shiny shoes?

They would add a name to my wardrobe: They are worth a lot of money at a fraction of the price.

The last point is the only one which did not only apply if they fitted. In fact, the chance of them fitting anyone was slight. If the shop had extolled the eBay benefit, they would have had so many more potential customers' attention. Other benefits did not fit the shoe. Even I wouldn't wear sparkly Jimmy Choos to the supermarket...often!

You need to find the right benefit for **your client.**

But first you need to find the benefits at all.

So ask yourself what does your customer *want?* What problem can you solve for them?

1. **For the doctor**: You save him valuable resources, time and money. You also improve his patient outcomes so you make him look good too. *He feels excited!*

2. **For the CEO:** you save him money in terms of covering absence. You improve worker productivity, and you improve staff retention figures, which also saves him time and money. *He is positively gleeful!*

3. **For the woman you meet at the gym**: You alleviate the probable course of why she has put on weight (and you save her time and money going to the gym). *She is ecstatic!*

4. **For the woman you meet at patient support:** You offer her the chance to feel listened to and an end to the frustration of looking for the cause of her stress. You also give her an opportunity to understand why she feels ill, rather than just that it is stress. *For the first time in ages she feels hopeful.*

So now you understand what benefits each customer is looking for you can start to build your pitch.

Some of these are generic for aromatherapy. Others you will have to find yourself, which are specific to your own practice and skills. Keep an open mind because your benefit for selling to a doctor will be different to a patient and different again to a large business or organisation.

Features of stress management as I see them, followed by their advantages.

Essential oil therapy
- Relaxing

- No side effects

- Luxurious

- Efficient

- It can be administered through massage but need not be,

- Able to continue using oils through week to improve outcomes

- Aromatherapy treats mental, emotional and physical all at the same time

- Enjoyable

- Feels like a treat

- Treatment is easy to follow

- Does not really need any will power

- There are a wide range of oils you can use so it is flexible

- Detoxifies and nourishes

- Clears pharmaceutical debris as well as fertilisers and petrochemicals

- Alleviates pain.

Other supporting therapies
- Help to get rid of the toxicity which is causing the physical manifestations

- Add to the efficiency of the aromatherapy.

One to one consultation
- Chance to have time to themselves

- Patient feels listened to

- Chance to focus on themselves

- Dedicated time to focus on getting them better

- Commitment to move forward from their problems

- Concerted decisions to try to get better.

Ongoing treatment
- Gradual foundation of slow steps forward is more effective than trying to go for the unrealistic quick fix.

- Allows them to make gradual changes.

Feedback and appraisal

- Rather than treating themselves alone: therapist is able to identify any set backs or opportunities to move things forward

- The patient is able to see developments outside of "are they ready to go back to work?" or "have my symptoms gone?".

- More chance of keeping up the therapy should they get despondent, rather than giving in before they give changes time to show.

Improvement in patient's mental outlook

- Helps them to see things can get better. Improved outlook alleviates stress.

Reduction in stress related symptoms
Self explanatory.

Improvement in general wellbeing

Improvement in productivity
I should add here that it is estimated that businesses payout **105 times more money a year** on presenteeism than they do in sick pay; that is on people who turn up to work and are too under par to do their jobs effectively.

Sales Benefits of essential oil therapies

1. Relaxing,

2. No side effects,

3. Luxurious,

4. Efficient,

5. Can be massage but need not be,

6. Able to continue using oils throughout the week to improve outcomes,

7. Treats mental, emotional and physical all at the same time,

8. Enjoyable; feels like a treat,

9. Treatment is easy to follow,

10. Does not really need any will power,

11. There are a wide range of oils you can use so it is flexible,

12. Can remove heavy metals and pharmaceutical debris.

Exercise:

Work out which of the list above can be turned into a benefit for

a) The CEO

b) The doctor

c) The lady at the gym

d) The patient

Tip: look back at what they want to achieve.

Corporate canvassing

Now my suspicion would be that most of you want to start ringing doctors first...that's where I would start too. But for the purposes of learning, understanding the company pitch is far simpler, then we can grow it.

You want to show that paying out your fee will save them time and money in the long run, otherwise there is no benefit to them buying.

Agreed?

So going back to your marketplace knowledge, pick the number which applies to your target. £476 for a private customer or £800 for public sector.

In the next chapter we will look at costing but for the purposes of this example I am going to say we are charging £50 a session because a set of 6 sessions would equal £300. Oh and by the way, for those of you outside London who just sat up in your seats and got very excited by £50, that's without your add ons like home treatments.

The business costs are:

- Sick pay - whether it is full pay or SSP. The company bears the cost until they can reclaim the SSP cost from the revenue *(find that amount from the tax office)*.

- The cost of replacing or outsourcing the employees work (would generally be the pro rata salary cost of the employee but also you can add an hourly rate of the person who has to speak to the agencies and interview for the post).

- The cost of possible employee support systems (average is £54 per person per year).

- Payroll costs: most companies use a company to process this - *you could probably find the cost of processing a payroll online*

Know your product

I have given you plenty of clinical data through each of my books, to use in your calls. Get used to talking about research into medical problems and couple them with aromatherapy's success stories. People want to know. The sources of the stats I have used in this book can be found in the bibliography at the back of this book (and the same applies for the other books too).

Open questions

There are two types of question. Use the right one and you will get great answers to move you forward, every time you make a call.

Open questions are designed to glean information. If you can remember back to school you will recall learning to write a newspaper article. All the answers to the open questions should have been in the opening paragraph.

They are :

Who, why, what, where, when, which. You kind of need to turn yourself into an inquisitive 3 year old.

Closed questions

Closed questions by opposition elicit yes and no. They begin with do you, would you, could you etc....These are useful on limited occasions but the open questions are king.

Getting past the gatekeeper

This might be the receptionist or the PA. Her job is to screen calls and keep the sales people out. There are two mistakes made here by rookies.

1) Underestimate her at your peril. A receptionist is never *just* the receptionist. She has the power to decide if you are worthy of the manager's time. It is her decision who gets to speak to her

boss. Respect her, and treat her well. It is only her key that will unlock the boss's door.

2) Do not try and sell to her. She may be an influencer but she has no money to spend. I'll cover this more in a moment.

As an aside, if she is a real Rottweiler and keeps you out forever you may need to play a little game. I often ask ""Lynn, I give up, the only way to get past you is to gonna be ring when you're on lunch. When are you going out to get a bite?" If you have done your job well and she knows you are serious about getting past her, she'll probably laugh and tell you.

Other reception blocks

We have a no names policy – Never mind, ask for one of the doctors straight off next time. They will tell you. Please don't abuse this. Doctors should be taking using their time making people well.

We don't take unsolicited sales calls – This one is harder. Get creative, pop some literature down to reception, find out who she is going to pass it on to and ask if you can follow up.

Maybe ring the commissioning unit at the Primary Care Trust, ask who the best person to speak to about requisition of third party referrals would be and ask if they mind you giving the practice a quick call....no longer unsolicited!

My point here is telesales is not hard but it can be incredibly frustrating. I could never list all the reasons you will not get through, but I promise you will if you persevere.

One last tip for any of you who catch someone on a really bad day and they hang up. Call back and say in your most saccharin of voices. I am so sorry, we got cut off, I just wanted to call back so you didn't think I was rude enough to do that on purpose.

In 20 years of selling on the phone only one person has ever owned up to hanging up on purpose and they gave me a 60K a year contract because they admired me for having the balls to bluff him on it!

Decision makers

Another thing you are going to have to be aware of doing is ensuring you are speaking to the right person. I say "don't canvass the cleaner". This goes for any sales call you do, whatever the capacity. You need to establish who is the MAN. That is who has the

- Means

- Authority

- Need

Does the person you are speaking to have the say so to make decisions and do they hold the purse strings? If they are not that person, we say they are an influencer and whilst these are very useful for gaining information ready to sell to the MAN, there is no point actually trying to get an appointment with them with a contract. Their signature is not worth the paper it is written on.

Ok so we will start with a sample script where things go relatively to plan. Watch for open questions and see where I use closed questions. See how I ask open questions to get info and closed questions to get yes or no answers.

B2B

Good Morning Tesco's

Good morning, can you tell me please who is the person to speak to, about staff sickness in your company?

Mary Portas

Thank you put me through please.

Many Portas,

Ms Portas, thanks for taking my call. I understand you are the best person to speak to about staff sickness figures in your business is that correct?

Erm, kind of I suppose. In what way?

My name is Elizabeth Ashley and I'm calling from thesecrethealer.co.uk, we are an aromatherapy provider specialising in stress management. I was hoping to find out a little bit about what happens in your business if a staff member is signed off with stress. Is that something you can help me with?

- I suppose first I should ask whether you have anyone signed off at the moment?

- When was the last time it happened?

- And how often does it happen there?

- How many employees do you have on site?

- I know research shows that shift workers are often the most vulnerable people to the effects of stress, is there any section of your business which struggles more than another?

- Drop in: *It's difficult isn't it because often people don't want to own up to stress and so they say the problem's something else. I know, the figures are pretty much impossible to be exact. Close is good enough.*

- How long does the average sign off last? Was that the longest?

- Have you had any staff actually leave that you think might be down to stress?

- What are staff absenteeism figures looking like for you at the moment? How does that compare to 12 months ago, do you think?

- Any idea what that might amount to in monetary terms for *your* business? I suppose you have to think about the cost of replacing their work through an agency or cross training, sick pay, payroll costs and of course they continue to accrue holiday pay during their sickness too, don't they? (Deliberately closed question: If she says yes, fantastic, you know your magic number, if she says no, potentially she will feel vulnerable and be interested to know yours – which is an average statistic of £476 in a private company, in case you can't remember).

- I know companies who have awards like IIP (Investors In People) have to benchmark the wellbeing of their staff don't they? What strategies do you have in place to benchmark and reduce stress in your business?

- You seem very clued up with your figures. Is your own job monitored against managing absenteeism?

In the following script I have tried to show the different scenarios you face so they don't trip you up when you come to them. It does make the beginning of the script repetitive but these are good habits to learn.

B2D

Reception: Mill Health Centre

Good morning, Can you tell me please, the name of the person to speak to about third party referrals for stress patients?

Reception : Dr Shepherd *(Not that I could speak for drooling if it was McDreamy but go with it!)*

Thank you. Put me through please. (Note: this is not a question. Take command)

Shepherd!

Dr Shepherd, thanks for taking my call. I understand you are the best person to speak to about the possibility of getting onto your list of approved third party referrals for stress patients. Is that correct?

No, actually sorry that's not me. You need to speak to Jac Nailer.

Oh ok, thanks for that. Jac Nailer Ok, got that, so who is she?

She is head of medical buying for our practice.

Ok that's great, I'll give her a call. Thanks for that, you've been really helpful.

New Call

Good morning Mill Health Centre

Oh yes hello, it is Elizabeth Ashley here again from thesecrethealer.co.uk. You very kindly just put me through to Dr Shepherd about third party stress referrals?

Yes

Yeah, he suggested I speak to Ms Nailer, I wonder, can you tell me, is she free?

No I am afraid she's not at the moment

Ah Ok, can you tell me when might be a good time to call?

She is usually free for calls between 3 and 5

Thanks that's wonderful, You've been really helpful. Sorry. What was your name?

Anna

Thanks Anna you've been great

New call

Good afternoon Mill Health Centre

Anna, it's Elizabeth from The Secret Healer again, you mentioned Jac Nailer might be free about this time. Is it possible to speak to her?

Yes, I'll just put you through

Thanks

Ms Nailer

Ms Nailer, I wonder if you can help me, I was speaking to Dr Shepherd earlier about how I could go about getting on the approved suppliers list for third party providers for stress. He suggested you might be the best person to help me. Does that sound right to you?

Yes, but I am sorry I'm too busy to speak to you at the moment

Of course, I understand. I'd love to call you back. When would be a good time for you?

Sometime next week.

That's great are you in on Wednesday about this time

Yes fine.

Thanks I'll speak to you then. Thanks for that

New call- Wed 3pm

-Good afternoon Mill Health Centre

Jac Nailer please.

-Who's calling?

It's Elizabeth Ashley from The Secret Healer. We have an appointment to speak.

-Nailer

Ms Nailer thanks so much for taking my call. You suggested that I call back today at 3. Is this a better time?

-Yes, if you are quick.

So what I was looking to find out is:

How you choose your third party providers?

.....

Is there a set system of referral, for example do you all refer to CBT or does each doctor have his own preferences?

....

What methods of healing do you tend to refer to? (Is it always counselling?)

.....

At a guess how often would you say you refer people for stress related conditions?

......

Gosh that is a lot. I'm surprised. That's a lot of people taking up your time, what sort of percentage of the workload would you say that was?

.....

How effective does it seem to be on the whole for your patients?

....

That's great to hear / That's disappointing, (depending on the response.)

.....

And what is the most important thing you look for from your providers?

......

What sort of follow up and liaison do you require from them? Do they submit case notes etc?

....

And how did you choose them in the first place?

.....

Potentially they will say they were told they have to use them by the Primary care or PCT, but that's Ok. You are information gathering here.

I'm guessing a large percentage of those will be for somatisation, is that right?

(ooo- hear the tone of her voice change, that's not an airy fairy hippy word...its an expensive budgetary expenditure word. You just got credible!)

....

What sort of size of problem does that represent in your practice? Gosh that's huge.

....

It's a shame there is no standard strategy for these people, isn't it?

....

How would I go about getting on to the preferred suppliers list?

.....

Who would I need to speak to?

Softly, softly, catchee monkey!

Can you see how they are very direct questions but I have softened the way I ask them. This is a really aggressive sales call but with a gently, gently approach. Always make sure your questions are not too pointed, but pointed enough to get the answers you need. The more you know about the business and processes when you come to sell back to them, the more powerful your pitch will be.

Incidentally, many sellers will come back with a benefit every time someone offers up a reason they might buy. I don't do that. I like to stockpile all mine for a massive attack. It works for me. You might find another way works better for you. It doesn't matter how you do it as long as you keep in mind...benefits, benefits, benefits.

One last thing, sometimes I won't sell back at all in that first call. I will ask if they mind if I call back next week. I tell them I want to take some time to assimilate all of the information they have been kind enough to give me to see if there *is* a way I can properly help or not. You would be amazed how effective being blasé and playing a bit hard to get can be.

A bit of wisdom from my first sales manager – You can't lose a customer you never had. No need to rush, or even worry about being too pushy. Converting a new client takes what it takes.

Happy with your info? Let's start selling back.

The Secret Weapon
I have a favourite question which I use in every sales scenario I find myself in.

"What is the Most Important Thing you are looking for? [From your treatment, from your provider, from your solution].

On my ratio monitor notes attached here, I write this as MIT.

Once you know their MIT you will be able to ascertain which part of your pitch you need to weight the most. Is it reliability, service, that they feel better, or is it price? Sell your solution to their MIT every time you speak to them. They won't remember they told you and it will seem like you have crept inside their head.

Very powerful, and this, people, is sales at its very best.

Right, when you feel like you know everything you need to know to build your pitch, start to tell her about your business:

"Ok good. So if I quickly tell you a little bit about the service I provide you can tell me if it is something you might, _in principle,_ be interested in.

As I said I am a clinical aromatherapist and stress is my specialist area. By that I mean not just using essential oils for relaxation but also treating the underlying issues and the presenting pain.

Usually clients come to me for a six week set of appointments each for an hour. In the appointment sometimes I will use massage but that doesn't suit everyone so often I will put the oils they need into creams and lotions. This means they also have ongoing medicines throughout the week between treatments. We look at how their diet could be making them worse, and get involved with basic lifestyle changes like taking exercise or some visualisation techniques. This gives the oils a chance to start working on their demeanour and their pain, but also generally helps to reframe their thoughts as well as detoxing their body.

So for many patients this works really well because they really feel more listened to. This is particularly true for those categorised with any sort of somatisation diagnosis. They get really good results by addressing their emotional issues rather than coming from a standpoint of pain. It empowers them to take control of their situation rather than simply focusing on their symptoms. Of course there are the added benefits of hopefully engaging them in healthy, more rewarding, lifestyles, especially with exercise and their diet.

I am not sure if you know that essential oils haven't got any side effects, only main effects, and since they are working with a qualified therapist it is a safe and effective way forward..."

All of this sits well in both pitches and then all you need to do is sum up your benefits to your client.

For the doctor:

"and of course hopefully it gets them out of your waiting room too. It frees up time for you to see more of your patients, so I am guessing it moves some of the budgetary issues too.

How does that sound to you?"

For the Personnel Manager:

"Of course the thing is this process helps them to be more resilient too, so not only do they get back to work more quickly which saves you money, but they are also taught to be more resilient to the rigours of their job which reduces the chances of them being signed off with stress again.

Not only does the process save you time and money but I have good enough paperwork for you to use it for evidence when applying for awards like IIP too."

Building a staircase of approval

What this means is stacking up the "yes"s. So, if I could free up some workload time for you, would you use my services? Yes. If I could take 10% of the "Time waste workload" away from you, would you buy? Yes. If I could assure you it was safe and has no risk for you, would you buy? Yes. If I could show you an audit trail if you needed to check anything, would you buy? Yes. Every time you take a "No, I would not buy, because" away from him, the more likely he is to buy. He is climbing your staircase of approval.

I almost can't speak without using the term "How does that sound to you?" because I have found people really answer it well. "I don't think it will work for me because..." "It sounds ideal for us because ..." or my very favourite one "Sounds like a plan!"

Kerching! Sold!

Is it starting to seem easier?

B2C

I hope really I shouldn't have much to teach you about selling face to face to individuals. You should have it down on pat. But here are a couple of pointers.

Open questions are still your best friend.

- How long have you had the symptoms?

- What are your symptoms?

- How do you feel?

- What do you feel stress is stopping you doing?

- What have you done so far to try to feel better?

- What does the doctor say?

- What medication did he prescribe?

- What oils have you been using yourself?

Now the last question would seem to point to a weakness in your pitch but of course it is your strength. Whilst they may be feeling more relaxed I would be very surprised if they have attempted to deal with the underlying toxicity or the spiritual disease. If you have genned up on *The Professional Stress Solution* you will be able to explain to them how, working together, you will be capable of so much more.

Sell on Service

Right then guys and gals, what happens if someone tries to knock you down on price?

Well, first of all congratulations on getting a fee at all. I find once people have been your case history model whilst you were training, they suddenly don't want to pay. This is another benefit of putting your business on a more commercial setting. They have a pot of cash; you simply have to get them to open it.

Negotiating on Price

Every day you will have someone who questions your pricing. It helps to remember it is not necessarily because they think your product is inferior but more because they want to feel good about how well they did getting a bargain.

From that you can deduce two things:

- First: it is not anything personal about you or the service you are selling.

- Secondly, and what many people don't realise: it is a buying signal. They would not be thinking about you reducing your price unless they were thinking they may want to buy it.

The second point is important because you need to remember you come from a position of strength. You have the product they want.

It is important then to decide very early on whether you, as a business, negotiate on price. Then, make it a rule and stick to it.

If the answer is yes then you need to build a haggle margin into your prices. Sometimes you will get lucky and your margin will be great, others you will have to reduce and your margin will just be OK.

OK is good, just be careful you do not trade at a loss.

If the answer is no, you will not negotiate on price, you must be prepared to be able to justify your price.

Think about this when you are doing your FABs. If they are not in there yet add them in.

- How many therapists are able to treat at such a deep level?

- Good results will get their patient/ staff member out of the doctor's waiting room and back at their desks.

- You have fully paid up insurance for their safety.

- Essential oils are not cheap commodities.

Think of every reason why you came to the figure and deliver it like a pro.

Then if that does not work...use mine!

An extremely pompous woman questioned how much I charge for my writing recently and scoffed she could get a contractor in India for half the price.

So, I pulled up as tall as I could, put on my bourbon sweetest smile and said,

"The thing is madame, I am fully aware of the market place value of my skills and the quality of the products and services I deliver, and I price my business accordingly. I can only surmise your Indian lady does exactly the same thing."

Not particularly pleasant but...match point to me!

My point is - do not be bullied. Your therapy has got to put bread and butter on your table and you have really got to fight for it.

Say the price and shut up!

Too many people get into the habit of sounding apologetic for their prices. Worse still they immediately add "but..." ready to open the floodgates to cutting their fees.

How often have you said "I charge £25 for half an hour, but..." You might swallow it but for many people it definitely is there.

If you are really gifted you could practise getting an intonation in your voice that says it's ONLY that much. Can you believe it?

My dad was a second hand car salesman and he used to tell me the first one to speak after the price was out in the open had lost the sales negotiation.

Do not be scared of the silence...let them think, because they are weighing up how much they want it. What's more, if they didn't have any interest, they would not have asked the price. See? You have the power!

The only reason a seller speaks after stating the fee is to offer some excuse as an apology for the price. Don't do it! Your customer's comment however, will help you to close the sale.

- That's expensive - Reiterate to them again. Why it is worth the price.

- I'll have a think about it – Think about what? What part have you not convinced them about well enough?

Get confident in asking that question, "Which part of it do you need to think about?" You can flip a conversion over in a couple of seconds after that.

Add Value

Whilst your customers may love the idea of aromatherapy the truth is that people only really buy from *people* they like. Build a rapport with them and offer them added value in their sale. Think about what works for you.

Adding value to a product or service means you give them more bang for their buck...and more importantly means you don't need to haggle on price.

Some ideas are

- Free gift of a bath oil

- Loyalty card

What are you offering that sets you apart?

Finally, now you are seasoned in really working the features and benefits of your products, you are overcoming objections like an Olympic steeplechaser and justifying prices comparable with the Manchester City FC physio bill, all you have to do is get the money out of their greasy paw! Piece of cake.....

In fact it really is like taking candy from a baby. Just remember this is where you use your closed questions.....

I'll just pop you in the diary for Monday at 4pm, shall I?

Can I have your email address to confirm your booking?

Or using an open question would be...

When would you like to come? (For an appointment! Rude!)

However you do it, there really is just one rule...

Ask for the sale!!

One final, final tip

Asking for the sale

Does this ever happen to you? Sometimes you know how you know something in one area of your life, but it doesn't always translate to another?

When I was a recruitment consultant I had a very high placement success rate, but that did not happen from the beginning. Then I asked one single question that turned it all around. I asked "What made you choose Dennis over Rosemary, to give him the job?"

As far as I could see Rosemary was a far better fit in every way for the role. So why had the client declined to offer her the position?

Do you know what the client said? "She never asked me for it so I didn't think she was that interested". No, no, no, no, NO! What a mistake-a to make-a! I never even thought to remind my candidates to ask for the job. From that moment on, I talked to every candidate about doing it and I think that single tactic improved my success rate by 50%.

If you want the business, *tell* the client you want the business. Even ask what you have to do to get the business if you want to. I do! "What would I have to do to get this deal?" Reduce your rate, buy me lunch, or take me to watch the Wolves game. I've had them all; including a few that would make you blush. Some I did, some I didn't. The point is, I put the power in my own hands. It became my choice whether I made the deal.

What's more, always let the client know *why* you want the deal, because who wants to buy from a supplier who does not feel excited by their agreement?

In ghost writing I do this a lot. A lady recently asked me to write something about an Ayurvedic medicine procedure called oil pulling. What's more she didn't want to pay a lot. Since I know nothing about the procedure I wrote back and explained very honestly about writing my own complementary medicine books, but knowing nothing about oil pulling at all. If she had source material for me to use, then I could write the piece. I explained that I could do a lower rate because she was in effect paying me to learn a subject where I have a weakness in my knowledge. I got paid for reading really! How great is that? Moreover, she knows I am likely to use her data and because I have been open she is happy for me to do that.

Think about the flip side for a minute so we can test the point. How annoyed do you get when you have been on hold to a call centre for an hour, to get someone who sounds entirely disinterested to hear from you on the other end of the phone. Worse still the woman on the checkout who is moaning to her friend about how long it is till her break. I know what I say - "I've a good mind to take my business where it will be appreciated!" How about you?

Effervesce to people, sparkle and be interested in getting that business for goodness sake! I promise you'll be stunned at the difference it makes. Who knows you might even find the sparkle catches and you find you love the thrill of the sell, because as far as I'm concerned it is one of the most fun things I've ever done. Don't believe me? Just wait till these tools turn your first sale then come back and answer it again!

A good deal means you get what you want as well as they do. Always remember that. If you are not earning enough or the client is not getting enough for their investment then that is a deal gone sour. Think about what you need, and what you are prepared to offer to get it. Quid pro quo.

And so the cycle continues, add value, sell benefits...because that is how the world works.

Overcoming Objections

Anyone new to sales is scared of objections. Anyone good knows they are a person thinking about buying out loud.

Let me put it into context. As I write, my husband is painting the kitchen (I know, I have so got this sussed!) We discussed paints. I wanted a yellow one.

- Objection – They don't do kitchen and bathroom in that shade.

- What about that one?

- It'll clash with the shade of the hall behind it.

- This green one's nice.

- Your orange knife handles will clash.

- Can you move the knife rack onto the white tiles on the plain wall?

- Yes.

- So the green will work then?

- Yes, let's go with the green.

There are two points to be made here. Had I sold all the benefits of green properly first, I could have made my life easier because he would have no objections to raise.

I should have said: it will go with the hall, it has the mould guard in so it will sort that problem too. If we put the knives on the other wall it all goes together.

The second is to show how if someone raises an objection they are simply trying the idea on for size....think of it a bit like "Does my bum look big in this?" They are visualising your plan.

If you can feed them the right benefit back, then you will very easily overcome their objection. Just take a deep breath and think about what you missed in your pitch. If you want to be as cheeky as I would be and ask the prospect.... "Let me ask you then, what would it take to make you buy?" You'll find out one of two things here, your sticking point, or the fact you might be talking to a person who is *never* going to buy. Not everyone wants your product, not everyone needs your product...you never know he could be sleeping with an aromatherapist! In which case you are probably wasting your breath!

Learning to Pitch

If any of you know anything about cricket, you will know you have to swing your bat and hit a very hard ball. The question is, how does a bowler find ways to get the ball past you to hit the wicket? The answer is, he varies his approach.

I never want you to go into a room and pour out a minutes worth of jargon at a customer. You should always go in with a consultative sell. In other words you are fact finding and then selling them back with their relevant benefits. This never changes. We simply need to find more and more ways to do this in a manner that fits your business. Yes, you can telesell, see people at shows, and even give presentations and talks.

We talked about the miserable wives whose husbands are affecting their weight. Remember where you might find them? We said spas, weight clubs, gyms, even counselling. Let's consider how you might approach doing a talk at a weight loss club. Incidentally here, I should say, groups are always looking for speakers. This is a great way to advertise your service to several people at one time.

So what's the biggest benefit to someone at a weight loss club?

I'm not going to answer it. You know.

What could we call our talk?

What about: Is being miserable making you fat?

Or : Is arguing more than just a weight on your shoulders?

And: Husband/ Partner! I've really had a belly full of this!

Those of you who struggle to make the associations between stress and weight gain, visit *The Professional Stress Solution* to fill in the blanks.

Talk about the science, then regale the features, advantages and benefits of your aromatherapy service and practice.

Get yourself properly prepared. Project your voice, have some interesting hand outs and you will have them in the palm of your hand.

One final exciting point is that many groups will pay you a fee for your time. Make yourself entertaining and interesting. It is rare for someone to speak big fat science at these sort of events. Knock 'em dead, get your fee for presenting, bookings for your clinic and I bet you will have requests for more talks too.

Of course there is nothing to stop you arranging a talk off your own bat too.

Closing the sale

Check out ads for companies looking for sales people. "Powerful closers wanted". Everyone wants someone how can clinch the deal. Want to know how to close this sale?

"When shall I book you in?"

End of lesson.

Chapter 4 Know your numbers

When I worked for Jill Bruce Aromatherapy, they sent me on a business excellence course. One of our seminars was given by a guy who sold private jets, cold calling from a telephone book.

Surprisingly he was rich...and I mean seriously rich.

He taught me the sales mindset and this is a very powerful thing.

He knew when he sold his jet the sale was worth £100,000 (that's how long ago it was!). He knew he would have to make 20,000 calls to find that buyer. Therefore each call he made was worth a £5. So he would write down the name of the person on his callsheet and he would tick every time someone said "No" and he would say "thank you very much, that's another £5 earned". If you can think about the journey when you are selling, rather than the destination, selling becomes a whole lot easier.

Now my conversion rate is much better than 1 in 20,000 mainly because my product is much easier to sell. I would suggest when you start to call you might have to make 10 calls to get through to a decision maker (because of reception blocks, it's their day off etc), then be able to get an appointment with 1 in 20 of them. That's not so hard is it?

What I will say is I have sold many different things, from recruitment solutions to packaging supplies and vending machines. The secret is practice. No matter how many years experience you have, those first few calls can be close to painful. Do role plays, talk to the mirror and expect things to go wrong....but know you will get better, and fast!

I use a manual ratio monitor sheet for my calls. Even after years of using computerised CRM systems, this works the best I think. It is a simple chart. You can download it from buildyourownreality.com/ratio-monitor for your ease. There are no frills, all you have to do is put ticks in boxes and add them up. For ease here, it looks like this:

Ratio Monitor Sheet

Name of prospect	Rec block	Inf	MAN	Notes	Follow up

It is fairly self explanatory. When you have finished your call, decide how to categorise it and put a tick in. At the end of the week you will be able to see how effective your calls have been.

A reception block is self explanatory, they stop you speaking to the MAN somehow...he might be on lunch or not in for the day or you may be politely told to get lost.

Be truthful about whether you have spoken to an influencer or not. If they gave you any information which moved your enquiry along, then potentially they were an influencer. Dr Shepherd was, he told us who we should correctly be speaking to. Ms Nailer potentially was, depending on the answers to her questions. If she decides who the practice refers patients to, then she is the MAN, but if she says the PCT does the buying, then she does not hold the purse strings and she is an influencer.

Remember don't canvass the cleaner. Ask for as much information as you can get from the person on the phone but unless you can prove they have money to spend, DO NOT Sell.

The ratio monitor sheet is primitive and it's boring, but it works. It is very easy to con yourself you have been selling all day only to find you have only done ten calls. Don't feel guilty, we have all done it. Just stop doing it! When I was a telesales manager I would expect my people to make 100 dials out a day. Really, I think if you can get 20 dials out and speak to two good solid decision makers, as well as seeing your clients, every day, you will have more business than you know what to do with.

I use index cards to keep a note of the progress of calls with each client, and I have a diary to log when the follow up call should be. I try to make a habit of calling 10 new prospects I haven't spoken to before each week.

Understanding conversion ratios

Whilst these will not give you a definite figure of your future business, they are a pretty good crystal ball. In theory, the better you get at selling, the more effective your conversions become.

If I make 100 calls a day, and I get through to 20 decision makers: The MAN conversion is one in five- 1/5

If I speak to 20 decision makers and I set up 2 visits to sign contracts: My visit conversion is 1/10

If I get one signature from those visit my conversion rate is one in two - 1/2

So I know then if I want to get 3 new corporate clients on board I need to go on

3x 2 visits = 6

Which will take me 60 calls to decision makers, which means I will have to do 300 calls in total.

Converting market share

So how many customers *can* you expect to convert? Since there are so many variables, such as how good your sales skills become, whether you pitch your pricing right, how receptive prospects will be to your ideas in your particular geographical location, it is very hard to say. In fact really there is only one projection I *can* accurately make.

If you don't sell, you will not grow your business. I have constructed that sentence carefully too, because I think you should be controlling how your business grows, not just expecting it to happen. Are you nourishing your little seedling with lots of new fresh opportunities or are you draining the lifeblood by churning out the same stuff over and over again?

Of course if what you feel I am telling you is s**t, just watch how the businesses who *are* using it start to bloom. I promise you life will be very rosy for them. The question is how will you even know if they are using it? Well the answer is of course, you should be watching.

Chapter 5 Creating a product to sell

This might be the shortest chapter in history because you should have plenty of ideas of your own. *The Professional Stress Solution* is a six week treatment plan involving massage and home treatments. This will of course be the most effective thing to sell. It will give you excellent results and is the best solution in the market. You can afford to charge what you like. It might not, however, be the easiest product with which to get your foot in the door.

How about offering to give a department a demonstration of hand massages to relieve the pain of RSI (I'd snap your hand off for that right now!). Foot massages for care workers. Back massages for office workers in their chairs. In the shopping centre, what about facials, or Indian head massage or whatever you want to plug. The main thing is you get people in front of you, a captive audience if you like, and tell them, even better show them, what you can do. Cost these events effectively so you can give a truly attractive deal. Get in the door and perform like your life depends on it, because in fact it just might do!

Think about the returns you could get on your fees. Could you offer an afternoon for a fixed rate fee? If so, be clear about how many people you are prepared to treat.

Think about talks you can give, presentations you can do and put yourself a portfolio together that sell, sell, sells.

Home Treatments

I am pretty sure all of you will have learned this in your diploma, but I am covering bases just in case. At every opportunity, upsell. The beauty of aromatherapy treatments is that home treatments do effectively improve your outcomes, so this is a very easy sell.

Ensure you are making body lotions and bath oils for your clients to use at home. Home in on opportunities of their birthdays to make them bespoke gifts. Every person who uses one of your products is a potential client to be had. Price these in a way they are profitable for you, but a present of choice for your clients.

Chapter 6 Tools

Competitor Swot Analysis

How much do you know about your competitors?
Do you know who they are? Do you even care?

We may have another one of those *sales person v
gentle soul* dichotomies again I suspect. I don't
know, so I'll ask the question. How competitive
are you? I'm not sure it is given as a standard in
a person spec for a healer. Do you want to be the
best and have all of the business available, or do
you feel more comfortable with the idea that
there is plenty of business to go round? Both are
fine, neither is better than the other as long as
you know that if you have someone like me on
your patch, your business is going to be
completely sucked dry if you are not on the
lookout for them.

The other reason for competitor awareness is to
learn what is happening in the marketplace and
respond to it. You would be amazed how trends
and patterns change. What's more if you know a
person's weakness you can make it your
strength, which is very exciting until you think
the predatory sales person will also have swotted
you.

So what is SWOT ?

We look at

- Strengths

- Weaknesses

- Opportunities

- Threats

Pick three businesses who you feel may be competition and do one on them. First though, do one on your own business.

I have taken some excerpts from the template I use myself and you can find this on a website called businessballs.com if you want it too. Basically though, draw yourself a big plus sign and allocate the four corners as strengths, weaknesses, opportunities and threats. By looking carefully at the whole picture of what is going on in your business at any time you will be able to see where you can jump on a chance which may not otherwise have come your way: Has one of their favourite therapists gone off to have a baby, have they started to market in a different way, how is their face book page doing, have they had a refurbishment? If you are in business, you simply have to know these things. I would suggest doing the first four, then doing one a month after that. Rotate the same ones or find new ones emerging who might affect your business.

- Capabilities?

- Competitive advantages?

- USPs (unique selling points)?

- Resources, Assets, People?

- Experience, knowledge, data?

- Financial reserves, likely returns?

- Marketing - reach, distribution, awareness?

- Innovative aspects?

- Location and geographical?

- Price, value, quality?

- Accreditations, qualifications, certifications?

- Processes, systems, IT, communications?

- Philosophy and values?

- Market developments?

- Competitors' vulnerabilities?

- Technology development and innovation?

- Global influences?

- Niche target markets?

- New USPs?

- Tactics: eg, surprise, major contracts?

- Obstacles faced?

- Insurmountable weaknesses?

- Loss of key staff?

- Seasonality, weather effects?

- Gaps in capabilities?

- Lack of competitive strength?

- Reputation, presence and reach?

- Financials?

- Own known vulnerabilities?

- Timescales, deadlines and pressures?

- Cashflow, start-up cash-drain?

- Continuity, supply chain robustness?

- Morale, commitment, leadership?

- Accreditations, etc?

- Processes and systems, etc?

- Management cover, succession?

-

So how do you get that data?
Much of it you will know. But what about asking your clients when you call?

"I was thinking of going to find *myself* a new therapist, is there anyone you can recommend?"

What about canvassing the businesses and clients: "Are you speaking to any other therapists about this kind of service at all?"

"Just as a matter of interest how do their charges compare with mine?"

Like a few pages on face book, if you can bear the boredom start watching them on twitter. Daft as it seems....go get yourself a massage! I bet you are overdue!

Of course there is much to be said for the old adage – if you can't beat 'em, join 'em! Get over and talk to them. Explain what you are doing and see if you might be able to share resources and ideas. Networking with the right person can be a fantastic way forward.

I think it is worth pointing out too, just because someone is having success in a field, doesn't necessarily mean copy it. If your neighbour seems to have Indian Head Massage wrapped up, you might decide to take it off your sales literature and strengthen your detox pitch. Or you might want to discover why she is getting those patients but you are not. Is it price, does she market it through presentations, what? That's the power of these things they make you ask questions you wouldn't otherwise have done and probe deeper than you have done before.

With knowledge comes more than a little power.

One of my favourite tricks to use when I am pitching for writing is to use the key strengths of my competitors and turn them into weaknesses. Most of the big boys out there who charge similar rates to me are boutique providers who have many writers working for them. This is one of their main benefits to pitch, because it means their work gets done very quickly and customers get a fast turnaround. It is a strength. But when I always say "Unlike many of the very good boutique providers I notice have applied for your position, I'd like to reassure you your work will be written by an expert in the complementary medicine field. Your assignment will be completed by the same writer who submitted this pitch". Suddenly their strength may not look as strong as it did. Can you see how you could make it work?

Pricing

Again, I am probably teaching my granny to suck eggs...or whatever it is she was supposed to suck. But...are you making enough money? If no, why is that? Is it because you are not charging enough or because you are not seeing enough clients?

Could the problem be you *don't know* how much you should charge? By now your competitor analysis should be giving you an inkling how much everyone else is charging but are you offering the exact same product and does your business/life cost as much to run? Think back to my snotty retort in the section about overcoming price objections. If you know your skills and product are superior, charge more, but know how to back it up with your explanation on price.

There is more though. I do think therapy in London should cost more than it does in Hull. The clinic rent is higher, the cost of living is higher and the salaries of the patients are potentially higher too. Essential oil prices though potentially stay roughly the same and this is how new therapists get -into deep water with their pricing.

Let's do an exercise to see if you are charging enough.

We will need to set two prices. The first is your price for the individual client, and then you also need a price for the sources who will send you plenty of work, the doctors, the companies, the counsellors, for instance. The latter will be the lowest possible price you can charge for your items without making a loss.

There are three separate variables here.

- The price of your materials

- The cost of your labour

- The overheads of the business

Read those again to be sure you have grasped the principal. If you sell an appointment for a treatment without taking *all* of these into account you are trading at a loss.

Whilst it would seem to be guesswork in the main, there are good ways to work each section out.

Price of Materials

This is best done at the time of purchase, but it is easy to back track later. Every essential oil, carrier, and laundered towel, needs to be added in. So if you have paid £15 for 5ml of oil, each ml works out to £3. Get into the habit of calculating this and writing it on a chart so you check you are not being expensively opulent with too many blends.

The industry standard is 20 drops to 1ml of oil, but of course it's not bang on. Your viscous bottom notes will be less and the fast dripping top notes, so difficult to control, will have more. But 20 works well for this. A drop of this oil then is 15p

If you have 3 drops in a blend then it is 45p and so on and so forth. I'm going to suggest a synergistic blend with three drops of three oils so we have 9 drops for this example. £1.35 for oils then (Clearly if you are using rose or yarrow for instance, you will rework with higher numbers)

Carrier oil of macademia nut @ £3/100ml = 10 mls used = 30p

Sheets and towels laundered - liquitabs £6 for 33 = 18p

Couch paper £6.50 -30 uses (?) =22p

Case history notes paper = 2p

The cost of your labour

This is more subjective as it will depend on what you are prepared to work for. Keep in your mind that minimum wage is over £6ph and you have a standard of living you will want to sustain. Let's set your rate at £0ph because it is unlikely you will be treating patients on a normal 9-5 day. I suggest you probably work less.

Now you will want to break that down into how much that equates to per minute. I make that 34p per minute

So half an hour treatment then: £10

But the treatment also owes me wages for the time I **have spent doing admin, sales and marketing to actually attract the patient to me in the first place**.

I calculate this by studying how much time in a week I spend actually seeing clients and how much time I spend doing the rest of it. I spend

30 hours a week treating and another 10 doing support. So then the ratio of my time is divided 3:1. For every half an hour I deliver therapy, I also need to add a third on top for that support so that is 10 minutes:

So for marketing support it owes me another £3.33. So wages for the appointment is £13.33

Overheads

It helps to have an overview of what you have spent over a certain period of time. I do mine three monthly to tie in with my accounting quarters.

Add up everything you have spent on gas, electric, phone, stationery, petrol, rent, training, text books, start up costs, loan repayments, fairs etc whatever it has taken to run your business.

Mine comes to £150 a month, £450 a quarter. Now the tedious/fun bit, depending on what your mindset is.

How many trading days in that quarter? Let's say 65 for ease.

Divide 450/ 65 days.

Divide that by the amount of working hours in your day

Then by 60 to get your overhead per minute!

This comes to less than a 1p!

Now we took 30 minutes to deliver the treatment, plus we also know it owes me 10 minutes of marketing (because it was a third on top) so it now owes me 40 minutes of overheads at a penny each.

So in all this treatment costs me:

Materials   2.07

Labour   13.33

Overheads   0. 40

In total   £ 15.80

When you think that most therapists think charging £15 will cover all eventualities, you can see why so many people's businesses go by the wall. Don't just follow what everyone else is charging because....they may not have a clue either. Get smart, get richer.

Now, this figure £15.80 is the very least you can sell it for. This is what is called your bottom line. You will want to pitch your whole sale price a little above it. Most people will be looking to make a third here so I would suggest a number of around £20

Now if you imagine this will be your price for doctors, companies and other businesses to buy from you, you can see why your margin can afford to be lower. They will be bringing customers to you. What's more because the number of clients you will gain from one of these deals means you can also relax a little on your future marketing too.

If however you are selling directly to the public you will need to set a "retail" price.

Really you have done the hard work knowing your bottom line. I think most businesses would agree to look at working towards a figure which is double your bottom line. If you are going to make selling "wholesale" part of your business model you may want to ensure the difference between wholesale and retail is very attractive to the buyer without putting their customer off.

My treatment then could afford to retail at anywhere about £25. A quick look at my competitors selling a similar thing shows there is reasonable parity between my price tags and others. In fact, if I wanted to, because it my service of detoxification is very in depth,I could possibly afford to go anywhere up to £30

I want to stay true to my mission of giving individuality at a reasonable price and settle at £27.50

Don't copy my numbers, use your own to see if you can afford to undercut me or find ways to build in value and smash mine out of the water.

Profit
The larger the corporation, the more definitions and measures they have for profitability. Some give a return on investments, others on asset, and the list goes on and on.

Your business has one. It needs to **have more money coming into the business than it has going out**.

As the meerkat would say "Simples!"

But what if it is not? What if the money starts to decline and costs begin to go up? There are two things you can do. You can sell more or you can cut costs.

These sound like flippant statements but like every good thing, the genius is always in the simplicity. I worked with a very wealthy entrepreneur for a while and he taught me many things. One thing I always refer to is, he said "Take time to *work on* the business *not in* the business". What he meant was take time to take your overall off and think, how can I squeeze a bit more out of that? Could I reuse some bottles, if I took the laptop off standby at night how much would I save? If I looked at diversifying that range, what would happen?

Always have in your mind:

- How can I cut costs?

- How can I sell more?

If you always work to these parameters and every item is priced with these elements in mind, you will soon start to move into a position of profitability.

Terms and Conditions

This bit is my word of warning. I genuinely think the corporate customers are your best way to sell but please don't take too many patients from one client at one time. Remember the saying: don't put all your eggs in one basket. You only need to make one slip with that client and they could drop you like a stone. Whether you make a wrong move or a competitor comes and steals your gig, suddenly you could find a massive hole in your income. Make sure you have a balance of some corporate and some private, and a diversity of services you can offer.

Make sure too, when you canvass them you don't take any bookings without knowing their payment terms. Unlike your individual customers, they are unlikely to pay on the day. You will have to invoice and then agree to their terms. This is important to consider because it will affect your cash flow. 30 days is standard, 60 days is scary and 90 days....well, get the hell out of there. If you can get 7 days...well done you! Fantastic job! Try it and see.

Just like the price negotiations, they are likely to try to bully you on terms. DO NOT agree anything more than 30 days, unless you have a private income which can see you through. Imagine the impact on your business if they are late or even do not pay. Just like the rest of us, businesses get hard up too. Be absolutely clear what you are committing yourself to from the outset. Perhaps just start with one or more patients and then build up when you are happy the client will pay on time.

To ensure the swiftest conclusion of invoice queries, get signed contracts before you supply services and always, always, always get a purchase order number BEFORE you see your client. Remember ask for these things before you deliver your service, because that's when you have the most power. If you leave it till after the treatment, they will see a way out of giving you your pay.

That's the rule. Stick to it. Signed contracts and PO numbers, before you open a bottle of oil. No exceptions. Period.

Referrals and Testimonials

There are some marketing strategies which will cost you a king's ransom, advertising in the paper for instance. Others cost you less, social marketing for instance. The most powerful and cheapest advertising is that which takes the form of a reference or testimonial.

Always ask your patients to give you some feedback and be ready to take it openly. In the world of lies, damn lies and statistics some bright spark decided a person who is happy with their service will tell one person but an unhappy one will tell ten! You know what? If the electricity company hack me off I reckon I tell a good few more than ten! Catch your patient when they are happiest, just at the end of their treatment, and capture their joy. If they are happy for you to use it in your marketing it is a very powerful thing.

Creating literature that sells

Translating your ideas into leaflets and fliers is invaluable to gaining and retaining interest in them. I belong to that dreaded group of craft show shoppers called the leaflet collecting brigade. Seriously, it is like a disease! I get on the train home with almost empty shopping bags and a pocket full of paper.

These hours on the return journey are where I do my shopping, away from the pushchairs and the shoving crowds. I love to see the fascinating things people say about their work. I like to really absorb myself in their passion and their pictures.

We speak a language of dumbed down words and in a face to face sales pitch *awesome*, *amazing* and *brilliant* are about as good as it gets. On paper though, you have time to create a soliloquy of glorious descriptions and words. Get creative. Root out your thesaurus and really work your vocabulary hard. Use bullet points where you need them but really SELL your product. Explain, draw pictures with your words, sketch a vision for your client to really believe in...then make sure you can damn well deliver it.

Remember at every stage – FABS

What is the benefit? What will they gain? What can you do to make their life better?

I'd be daft not to add here.....if you are really rubbish (and incidentally you probably aren't) hire me to help! Details of how to do that can be found at elance.com/1st-Class-Contractor

Maslow's Pyramid

I had quite a tussle about which book this belonged in because it is important you understand it has applications in so many different realms for you. It is a well respected marketing tool, so it does sit well in this section. It is, however, also vitally important in how you gauge a person's transition through their therapy as well as a very useful self appraisal tool. I could have taken the choice to simply write about the sales and marketing applications, but I am also adding in some therapy aspects too. It doesn't really make sense under the title of the book, but I suspect every healer would be excited to discover it, so here goes....

I called this book *Sales Strategies for Gentle Souls* because I am aware of the quandary many therapists have. They are uncomfortable how the normal model of selling sits, and feel it has little integrity. I agree, spouting facts at a patient does nobody any favours. I do, however, believe you and I have very particular skills even the best double glazing salesman does not have. We have insights into human nature and we try to understand what makes people tick. This is a tool which will show you why having a foot in both of the healing, and the sales and marketing, camps is such a powerful thing.

Abraham Maslow was a psychologist who published his work *The Theory of Motivation* in 1943. He talks about people's needs as they go through life, with the most fundamental needs at the base of the pyramid and moving up. They stack up from the bottom like this:

Self- Actualisation

Self esteem

Social

Safety

Physiological

A person is only ever looking to fulfil a need which is one step away from where they are but will consistently look to keep safe the things they have already established. To explain that, let's flesh out the levels a little. To do this I am going to turn the pyramid of needs upside down so you can see the stages as they need to happen. So we start with physiological.

1. Biological and Physiological needs - air, food, drink, shelter, warmth, sex, sleep.

2. Safety needs - protection from elements, security, order, law, limits, stability, freedom from fear.

3. Social Needs - belongingness, affection and love, - from work group, family, friends, romantic relationships.

4. Esteem needs - achievement, mastery, independence, status, dominance, prestige, self-respect, respect from others.

5. Self-Actualisation needs - realizing personal potential, self-fulfilment, seeking personal growth and peak experiences.

Think of the worst states of society. If a person does not have food and shelter, they seem no longer to have a perception of danger in their hunt to feed themselves and lay down for the night. It is human nature to always build on these needs from the bottom and then work up. In fact, Maslow says that every person has the capability to achieve self-actualisation, but asserts only about one in a hundred people manage it. Many people get locked further down the pyramid.

In the 1970s his work was expounded upon and further stages were added into the pyramid. Self-actualisation moved from its position as step 5 and moved to 7. Inserted were

5. Cognitive needs - knowledge, meaning, etc.

6. Aesthetic needs - appreciation and search for beauty, balance, form, etc.

Then after it came a final step

8. Transcendence needs - helping others to achieve self-actualisation.

So the pyramid now looks like this

Transcendence

Self- Actualisation

Cognition

Aestheticism

Self esteem

Social

Safety

Physiological

So how does this help you with your sales and marketing?

Think about the adverts on the TV. Will a person who has financial worries be engaging in ads about cruises? No, they will be looking for loans. Does the cruise company care about that? Well, yes and no. They don't care about the person who needs a loan in any other way other than to strike them out of their target market, which is good for them because it helps them to narrow their pitch. Because they are no longer trying to sell to everyone they can pitch it somewhere around "Self Esteem". They are confident their target group is probably married couples who are happily in that slot, or perhaps divorcees who are in danger of feeling they are losing their self esteem and are anxious to get it back. Aestheticism is just above these people and so it is close enough for them to care about it, so the ad is completely focused on how lovely the cruise will be.

Marketing companies are absolute wizards at this. So much so that one of the reasons Maslow feels such a small percentage of people reach self-actualisation is most advertising pitches are sold at self esteem, so few people ever strive above it.

Let's put it into context by looking at where your patients might be in the pyramid. At a guess most of the ones who are under the doctor will be crushed at around/beneath the self esteem level. Those who are under financial pressures may be in danger of falling below that rung on the ladder. If you are pitching them benefits pertaining to self-actualisation, they will not buy. In fact they will not give a toss! Find ways to help a person onto the next rung of the ladder and you will engage them in your sale. What is important though is buying from you really will move them forward in life.

I am guessing you are shouting at me now, "But how do I know?" Use your open questions. Listen to the answers you get. Why not even ask those you speak to on a face to face basis "Do you feel like your basic needs are being met at the moment? Do you feel safe? How would you rate your self esteem?" If a marketing exec asked me that, I would think "You condescending little..." but coming from a healer, it has a very different note. I would be impressed at their compassion and empathy and the fact they wanted to know how I felt.

By contrast, even though you are selling the same product of a stress solution to a personnel manager or doctor, potentially their needs may have been met further down and they may be looking to move far higher. They are probably almost at transcendence and so talking to them about how they will be *helping* their staff member to move forward or develop will appeal.

Self-Actualisers

It probably is superfluous to reiterate the process of self-actualisation is one of becoming, rather than actually a ladder rung onto which we step. Of course it is. The same applies for every step. I like to think of it like an inkblot spreading, growing, blurring the lines. Slowly we become more of one thing and less of another.

Maslow made a study of 18 people, out of which he fashioned 15 indicators which he felt showed a person who had reached self-actualisation. How many of these would you say you had achieved? I never made it past number 1! I can tick quite a few others though.

Maslow lists the following characteristics of self-actualizers .

They have:

1. More efficient perception of reality and more comfortable relations with it
2. Acceptance (self, others, nature)
3. Spontaneity; simplicity; naturalness
4. Problem centering [as opposed to ego-centered]

5. The quality of detachment; the need for privacy
6. Autonomy; independence of culture and environment
7. Continued freshness of appreciation
8. Mystic and peak experiences
9. Gemeinschaftsgefiihl [a feeling of kinship with others]
10. Deeper and more profound interpersonal relations
11. The democratic character structure
12. Discrimination between means and ends, between good and evil
13. Philosophical, unhostile senses of humour
14. Self-actualizing creativity
15. Resistance to enculturation; the transcendence of any particular culture

Further he gives us some behaviours which will eventually lead to self-actualisation.

Concentration

"First, self- actualisation means experiencing fully, vividly, selflessly, with full concentration and total absorption". This is very "of the here and now" I think. There is a great deal of focus on mindfulness techniques around at the moment and I do think these are of a great deal of value. I think too, there is a great deal to be said for having a purpose in life and applying yourself to it.

I wonder how many of us really lose ourselves in total absorption. This is almost a childlike quality. How easy is that to invoke?

Growth Choices

I quite like how healthily this fits actually, because in the context of this book we can say - will you choose to grow into your newfound sales ability? Of course, the motivation can be two fold, can't it? Will you be motivated to move onward and upwards, or will fear of the unknown, or even comfort of the *known* be a bigger motivator to avoid this opportunity to move forward.

The same can be said for any choices, challenges or opportunities, how motivated a person is to take the step into the unknown will affect how much he or she is able to develop and grow.

Honesty

Those of you who have already read *The Professional Stress Solution* might have a wry smile here about the correlation with yin disease.... honesty with whom? At this point in development, a person has learned the skill of introspection and is able to be honest with *themselves* about challenges and issues that face them.

Judgment

With the ability to be honest with one's self, there comes an opportunity to be objective. This is the only possible way to exert truly good judgement.

Self-development

It fascinates me how some people with average abilities can turn these into something remarkable, yet others with remarkable gifts oftentimes achieve nothing at all. I wonder too how many people leave school and never try to learn anything again.

I can at least feel a certain sense of satisfaction in that I can tick this box and so I suspect can you. , though, are finding ways to look outside themselves and to spur themselves on? You might find Jill Bruce's work *Out of The Labyrinth* interesting here. Her book is entirely based on mindset and affecting your world through thought; no oils, no therapies, just thought. It is a very interesting read.

Peak Experiences

"Peak experiences are transient moments of self-actualisation" I like to think of these as the **whoopee** moments! Those, when the penny drops and you realise you just did something great. Those split seconds when your happiness makes time stand still; the rare moments when you are loved and feel loved and all is right with the world. At the top end of these we have the "Transcending self-actualisers" who feel these far more often than the norm. Or of course they may be taking something I have yet to discover, but I certainly would like some of that please!

Lack of Ego Defences

Here I write from my own place of weakness. As a very shy ghostwriter my gut reaction is always to hide. This is my own personal ego defence. In truth, I am completely aware I will not be able to develop properly until I find a way to get past that way of defending my ego. In fact this defence is one of the main behaviours that STOPs me self-actualising. We all have particular defences we put up. As they start to fall though, we move a little closer to our goal.

(*NB: well done Liz for your honest insights and intention to work towards this goal. As the wonderful CBT coach Sheila McMahon would say in her impenetrable Irish accent... "Now would you please get out of your own way!"*)

Chapter 7 Managing your Time

Because I am the world's worst at this, I do have some tips to share.

My top tip would be:

It's not what you know it's who you know...

One of the best ways to improve profitability is to use your time differently. That makes one of the basic tenets of my writing business. I'm good at writing, many people are not. What's more, if an MD of a company wants to spend 120 minutes of his £100 an hour salary writing something which I can potentially write in half an hour, it will cost him £25 to pay me or £200 to do it himself. Basic economics baby - if you think you can't afford an administrator, look at the maths again. If you were to spend that two hours treating someone, how much money will it bring you instead? If it is more than you will spend to outsource, your bank manager should be smacking you round the head.

Work *on* your business not *in* your business...do you know what the pennies are doing behind the scenes? Understanding your figures and perhaps having your accountant draw up some management accounts won't only show what your business is doing now, which bits are making the money-men smile, but also it will show you which taps are leaking resources and might potentially need shutting off. If you are scared of the numbers, have a look at Anna Goodwin's page on Buildyourownreality.com. Her books are designed to get even the biggest wusses out of their accounting hidey holes and you will grin right the way through them. They are great fun.

Procedures

Would you leave a load of 16 year olds in charge of a multi-million dollar corporation? It sounds like a disaster waiting to happen, doesn't it? Yet McDonalds do it every day. It works because everyone has a set system of procedures to follow and they emulate them without fail. There doesn't need to be much thought put in and should something go awry it is easy to pin point where.

I mentioned Investors In People in the sales pitches to companies. There are any number of awards these organisations will be pitching to win. The reason is, these prove they have strategies and procedures which keep their business framework in place. Manufacturing companies for instance boast of ISO 9001/2 or ISO14001, these show they have proven they have recognised practices of training, reporting, fault finding, invoicing, every aspect of their business is structured and transparent. 14001 is an environment accreditation which governs emissions and wastes.

If you see any of these accreditations on their website and then you turn up to a meeting without documentation of your procedures you will be kicked out of the door faster than you can say "Smell my lavender oil". You must be able to demonstrate an audit trail.

I have done some of this for you. The case history form in *The Professional Stress Solution*, your ratio monitor sheet, making your index call logs, having a transparent system of pricing and also having evidence of knowing where to go if you encounter a business problem (to re-iterate you can find my go-to people on Buildyourownreality.com. Please, use them. The longer they stay in business the better it is for me!) You might want to do risk assessments and health and safety policies – big companies positively salivate over documents as boring as these. In their supply chain, transparency is king. Anyone with 14001 will be looking for how you reduce your carbon footprint, and of course aromatherapy sits brilliantly here, talk recycling, sustainable oils, responsible care of waste. Embrace it....forget the scent of chamomile, you will be smelling profit all the way.

To thine own self be true

I have written scripts to help you, but repeat them verbatim and you will sound like a prawn! I speak with strange syntax so you really have to make the words your own. It's more than that though, I really don't want you to be a corporate clone.

Your healing skills are magical. You gravitated to that job because you are a completely extraordinary person. Let's face it, you make people better using plants! How incredible is that?! Please, don't think for a second I want you to change. Think of this training as another string to your bow, or another oil in your box. In fact yes, what oil could it be?

I know. Think of it like helichrysum. Its other name is everlasting, and this training will bring longevity to your job. It is an overall tonic, it makes everything better. So does having some money in the bank! Helichrysum vibrates on the throat chakra and so does sales. Agreed then? Think of sales like helichrysum. Work it into your business to make a synergistic blend.

Altering the slant of your business though, might mean things like your wardrobe needs to change. Think of the first impression you make if you go to pitch at the doctors dressed in overalls. You want to exude personality and drive, but you also want to be seen as a healer too. I would recommend you hop over to ByAriane.com (also found on my site) for her tips and techniques for getting corporate looks, which look individual but refined. What's more ladies I would be doing you a disservice if I didn't give you a heads up on her delicious bags...oh my goodness, the bags!

I believe very strongly we were all put here for a purpose. Each of us has a job to do. Our innate skills and qualities make us unique for the jobs we can perform. Perhaps writing these books was my purpose. I don't know. Perhaps we'll get to see. Last year I did some amazing work with Luanne Simmons of Goddess on Purpose, and she helped me a great deal with this. It took me a long time to find how all the pieces of my life history could come together and make something truly worthwhile.

I do have other skills. I can put a fish slice sideways in my mouth, but so far I haven't found a use for that. My daughter can put both feet behind her head and that is just as unsettling to see as the fish slice! You too will have talents and skills very few people have...hopefully a little less unsettling than ours. Can you find a way to channel them to give you joy and a new creative edge? If you find them I promise you the universe will do everything in its power to support you in your quest. Angie McKay's Wise Woman's Journal might help you to find your gifts. If you have not yet seen these extraordinary books, feel free to download a back copy at buildyourownreality.com/wwj-back-copy/

I have every confidence you can find a way to sell. Your own way...in a way that will bring you joy. I wish you success and profit and don't forget me when you make your first million!

Conclusion

I hope you are rubbing your hands in glee by the time you get here. I'll reiterate one more time, the first time you use these tools you *will* be next to useless! Don't be disheartened, I always am too. It is practice, practice, practice....

I am aware I have covered only sales, and marketing will be very useful too, so you may want to check in on "how to build an aromatherapy website that sells". Of all the marketing techniques you can learn, direct marketing will always have the best results. Don't be afraid of making the calls, the results will speak for themselves.

If I am honest, I am very nervous about the way aromatherapy is going, I can almost see it swallowing its own tail. It has reached a time when it could explode into a hundred different areas and make millions of people better. But at the same time the internet is inundated with pages upon pages of information about what essential oils can do, written mainly by people who have never treated a person or perhaps ever been near a bottle of oil.

I don't like treating people. Actually, I should rephrase that and say I don't like *meeting* people, and so therefore I don't like seeing people for treatments. I am however very good at my job. If I were to recruit you to train you to treat people for me...I'd have to meet you too. No offence, but that does me no favours either. Therefore...if you are a healer, *please* get out there and heal. Use my skills, take my knowledge and let's reverse the aromatherapy world on its axis. Let's get it back to a place where it is about getting people through your door onto the couch and getting them well. Let's have people qualified to sell oils doing it into the patient's hands. Most of all let's ride the wave of interest everyone seems to have in our art and get out there and push its talents as far as they can go.

There seems to be a trend in our community which says we should not make some money. It's almost as if some healers feel something has no integrity the second you pay for it. Perhaps those of you who have already read *The Professional Stress Solution* might attribute it to yin energy. Perhaps it is, I don't really know. All I do know is it is doing none of us any good. We pay extra for organic, because we know it is good. Why in the name of all that is good and pure, should you not be charging top dollar for your work. You have trained for years to do it, your materials are superb and you have a skill very few people have.

In short people...let's stop messing around and get out there and start making some money.

Other books by the author

Book 1 - The Complete Guide to

Clinical Aromatherapy & Essential Oils for the Physical Body

Essentially...essential oils for beginners, talented novices and intermediate aromatherapists

Let me ask you, why do you want a book on aromatherapy?

Do you want to learn how to care for your family naturally?

Perhaps you have a franchise selling essential oils and want to know more about what they can do?

Maybe you love the delicious scents and want understand how these beautiful things come to heal.

I wonder if you have started to learn and now want to discover how to build on your knowledge.

Whatever you are looking for this book has something for you.

- Details of how to treat over 60 conditions with essential oils
- Profiles of over 100 natural plant essences and their safety data
- Descriptions of 15 carrier oils and their applications not only for massage but also adding to creams and lotions.
- Comprehensive data of how the chemistry of an oil will affect its actions
- In depth insights into how professional aromatherapists blend...including their 13 favourite recipes from their practices.

Including....

- Sensuous aromatherapy blends by a qualified sex therapist
- Two blends for labour by the midwife running an aromatherapy program on an NHS maternity ward
- A blend for depression by a qualified mental health

PLUS....

10 bonus essential oil monographs and a complementary hypnotherapy relaxation download.

Discount vouchers of treatments courses and products by participating therapists.

AND.... for those of you who would like to contribute, there is a chance to make a donation to cancer research too.

This is my gift to you.

FREE - From 30.11.14

Book 2 Essential Oils for Mind Body Spirit
The Holistic Medicine of Clinical Aromatherapy

Healing the skin, easing the tummy ache or getting someone to sleep is easy with essential oils. Anyone can do it. The joy of healing, though, comes from peeling back the layers of the disease, almost like a detective to find out exactly what caused it in the first place.

Consider this book to be lesson 2 in The Secret Healer Series.

You have mastered which oil to use for what and why...this book takes you step by step though the ancient healing mechanisms of the aura, the chakras and meridians but also explores how that ties in with the latest scientific discoveries into how the emotions affect our health. Using Candace Pert's remarkable "Molecules of Emotion" research, The Secret Healer shows you *where* to look for healing links and *why*.

- Uncover how a certain recurrent negative emotion can be the trigger to make you ill?
- Understand internal processes that mean that psychology, neurology and immunology are quintessentially, and inextricably linked.
- Learn how to use essential oils control your emotions and in turn bring about a far greater standard of wellness.
- Discover mindblowing research that shows the emotions we experience are actually the sensations of neuropeptides triggering our organs to do their jobs
- Reflect on the wonder of Chinese medicine and ancient healing being completely accurate in their healing mechanisms for thousands of years...now that science proves it to be so.

Essential Oils for The Mind Body Spirit couples ancient wisdom with cutting edge science. This is the knowledge the drug companies hope you never find out and our doctors pray we all will.

A short write up, for a book that will change your life. I promise you, when you read the latest findings of psychoimmunolgy, you will never waster another day on being angry again.

The Professional Aromatherapist's Liver Detox

We are warned of the threats of heart attacks, strokes and cancer, especially if we are overweight.

What is kept quieter is doctors have established a link between toxicity in the liver and metabolic syndrome, the condition that leads to many of these conditions. What's more non fatty liver disease is known to underlie many other conditions such as eczema, allergies and headaches.

The scandal is just how many of our livers are struggling under the strain of over processed foods, pharmaceutical debris and actually even our own bad tempers!

This book explains:

- The importance of the liver and its functions
- How it becomes dysfunctional and how to interpret warning signposts
- How to cleanse and nourish using not just essential oils, but also vitamins and minerals and diet.
- The strange correlation between how our emotions translate negativity into disease.

- How to implement other therapies such as chiropractic, acupressure and counselling and how to secure fantastic referrals.

This book is best used in tandem with The Professional Stress Solution to benefit from the complementary healing. Use Sales Strategies for Gentle Souls to create a marketing plan to use your new found knowledge to smash your competition out of the water!!!

Book 4 The Professional Stress Solution
Essential Oils and Holistic Health Stress Management Techniques for The Professional Aromatherapist

Stress is pandemic in our society.

Scientists agree it plays a quintessential role in how likely it is we will suffer from chronic and possibly fatal illnesses in the future. Risk factors of metabolic syndrome, diabetes, stroke and heart disease are increased through stress.

The daft thing is....aromatherapy can do amazing things to ease it, and potentially aromatherapists could take a massive workload away from the doctor's surgeries.

- Discover the hormonal changes and peptide triggers that change a person's health and mental state.
- Learn how it affects the liver, adrenals and pituitary gland.
- Uncover the strange phenomenon of Yin disease
- Build a better foundation of care, but also a knowledge base that means you can sell your treatments more effectively.
- Improve your healing skills set
- Supercharge your referrals potential from other complementary therapists and orthodox medicine alike.

Includes free bonus material of

- Chiropractic chart of misalignments and potential organic disturbance
- Chart of the meridians and suggested acupressure points to detox the organs more quickly
- Detailed information about how to improve the patients condition with vitamin and minerals therapy
- In depth dietary advice
- Free hypnotherapy relaxation download

Essential Oils are The Off Switch for stress. The *Professional Stress Solution* is the ON SWITCH for your aromatherapy business.

Book 5 The Aromatherapy Eczema Treatment
Healing Eczema, Itchy Skin Rashes and Atopic Dermatitis with Essential Oils and Holistic Medicine

Most people appreciate that the itching and redness of eczema can be used using essential oils, but what if I told you they were capable of so much more?

Imagine if, as a therapist, you were able to pinpoint the emotions that set off these flares? Can you visualise what it would mean to your patient if you were able to isolate the very protagonist causing the eczema breakout and alleviate their pain completely?

Well now you can.

This book teaches you:

- How to isolate the emotions causing the emotional cycle of pain
- The likely food triggers for your patient and the tools to identify the exact times they will detonate a reaction

- The familial traits and links that lead to atopic eczema
- How these links connect with the liver and in turn how to cleanse the liver toxicity
- Vitamins and minerals to cleanse and nourish the system

The book contains very real that will not only transform the way you treat clients, but will skyrocket your clinic's takings.

I recommend reading this book in tandem with *The Professional Stress Solution* and the *Essential Oil Liver Cleanse* to fully understand the cycles and processes of treatment. Add to it *Sales Strategies for Gentle Souls* and your business will stand on an entirely new footing.

Why not save yourself 1/3

And treat yourself to the set?

The full and comprehensive course into how to heal eczema

with aromatherapy and essential oils I promise you...you won't regret it.

www.thesecrethealer.co.uk
www.buildyourownreality.com

Book disclaimer

by SEQ Legal

(1) Introduction

This disclaimer governs the use of this book. [By using this book, you accept this disclaimer in full. / We will ask you to agree to this disclaimer before you can access the book.]

(2) Credit

This disclaimer was created using an SEQ Legal template.

(3) No advice

The book contains information about sales training. The information is not advice, and should not be treated as such.

You must not rely on the information in the book as an alternative to legal or financial advice from an appropriately qualified professional. If you have any specific questions about any legal / medical / financial / taxation / accountancy matter you should consult an appropriately qualified professional.]

You should never delay seeking legal advice, disregard legal advice, or commence or discontinue any legal action because of information in the book.

(4)   No representations or warranties

To the maximum extent permitted by applicable law and subject to section 6 below, we exclude all representations, warranties, undertakings and guarantees relating to the book.

Without prejudice to the generality of the foregoing paragraph, we do not represent, warrant, undertake or guarantee:

    ⅄ that the information in the book is correct, accurate, complete or non-misleading;

    ⅄ that the use of the guidance in the book

will lead to any particular outcome or result; or

⅄ in particular, that by using the guidance in the book you will improve your business or guarantee profit.

(5) Limitations and exclusions of liability

The limitations and exclusions of liability set out in this section and elsewhere in this disclaimer: are subject to section 6 below; and govern all liabilities arising under the disclaimer or in relation to the book, including liabilities arising in contract, in tort (including negligence) and for breach of statutory duty.

We will not be liable to you in respect of any losses arising out of any event or events beyond our reasonable control.

We will not be liable to you in respect of any business losses, including without limitation loss of or damage to profits, income, revenue, use, production, anticipated savings, business, contracts, commercial opportunities or goodwill.

We will not be liable to you in respect of any loss or corruption of any data, database or software.

We will not be liable to you in respect of any special, indirect or consequential loss or damage.

(6) Exceptions

Nothing in this disclaimer shall: limit or exclude our liability for death or personal injury resulting from negligence; limit or exclude our liability for fraud or fraudulent misrepresentation; limit any of our liabilities in any way that is not permitted under applicable law; or exclude any of our liabilities that may not be excluded under applicable law.

(7) Severability

If a section of this disclaimer is determined by any court or other competent authority to be unlawful and/or unenforceable, the other sections of this disclaimer continue in effect.

If any unlawful and/or unenforceable section would be lawful or enforceable if part of it were deleted, that part will be deemed to be deleted, and the rest of the section will continue in effect.

(8)   Law and jurisdiction

This disclaimer will be governed by and construed in accordance with English law, and any disputes relating to this disclaimer will be subject to the exclusive jurisdiction of the courts of England and Wales.

(9)   Our details

In this disclaimer, "we" means (and "us" and "our" refer to) Elizabeth Ashley trading as Buildyourownreality.com, which has its principal place of business at 4, SY8 1LQ.

Acknowledgements

Top of the list in this book comes my dad. Sadly he passed away in Feb 2011. I miss him every day. Writing this book really made me feel close to him again I recalled all the things he had taught me about sales.

As a child he used to drive me mad. Whatever I asked him for, he'd have an argument why it could not be done; devil's advocate was his favourite game. He'd calmly make me go away and think my request out better for me to present again. I've been overcoming objections since I was four! The second hand car salesman had more integrity than anyone else I have ever known. His funeral was full of people who had bought every car they owned from him. They trusted his knowledge and knew he would tell them the truth. I hope people come to say the same of me.

Anna Goodwin, what would I do without you? Writing our books at the same time has been such a gift. Thanks for taking the time to bounce round ideas and always being there when I have wanted a moan!

Clare Ella, as ever, I thank you from the bottom of my heart for being a rock and eagle eyed proof reader of everything I write. You truly are an amazing woman.

To Kerry Collins, Dean Collett, Laki Bhamra, Julie Harris Tighe, James Ritchie, Laurence Reddy, Matt Wainwright and Gaynor Frost for everything you have contributed to my sales and recruitment knowledge. KC, who would have thought that first "Sell me this pen" would eventually lead to this? Aren't you glad to see "Go On" still has an effect!

To Rob of Robert Elsmore Images, for your wonderful representation of the Secret Healer on the cover.

To Jenine, just because! To Angela, also just because! I can't express how much you two faeries add to my life. To Richard, thank you for my peace of mind with IT and sorting out the buildyourownreality website for me.

To all my moms! My real one Jill Bruce, my step mum Pauline and my mother-in -law Pat, thanks for checking in on me and giving me the odd kick up the asterisk.

To Liz Thompson for reading my work...regardless! It means a lot.

To Tamara: for your help with the sick pay issues, to Ariane for the confidence boosts, to Faye for backing up Darrell's persuasion to start writing for myself and for our walks putting the world to rights during that wretched walk up the hill!

But most of all, thanks to my amazing family...my three children and husband.

To my daughter and elder son, away at university, thanks for giving me the space to write! Thanks for always letting me know what you are up to and letting me live so much excitement through your lives. I need to invent a new word to express how incredibly proud I am of you both. Middle man, thanks for all the pythons and php! Belle, your bravery inspires me so much; thanks for showing me life is so much larger than I once thought it was.

To the wee man, I hope you read this when you older so I can remind you how, at the age of 5 you lost two chapters of this book because you wanted to watch lego movie videos and you snatched the computer away! You are my little prince and I adore you. To my long suffering, always tidying up after me, complete rock of a man; through this book and every book you are wonderful and I thank you with all of my heart for choosing me to be your wife.

Bibliography

Beat Stress at Work. (2012, Jul 07). Retrieved June 28, 2014, from NHS Choices: http://www.nhs.uk/Conditions/stress-anxiety-depression/Pages/workplace-stress.aspx

HSE. (2010). *Managing health at work – recording and monitoring* . http://www.hse.gov.uk/research/rrpdf/rr310.pdf.

http://www.cipd.co.uk/NR/rdonlyres/22CB05C5-E52D-445B-891A-9886C95FD90D/0/absmgmnt0706.pdf. (2006). *Annual report survey*. CIPD.

Lansley, A. (2010, July 12). *Equity and Excellence, Liberating the NHS*. Retrieved June 29, 2014, from National Archives: http://webarchive.nationalarchives.gov.uk/20130107105354/http://www.dh.gov.uk/en/PublicationsandstatisticsPublications/PublicationsPolicyAndGuidance/DH_117353

Maslow. *(The Farther Reaches of Human Nature, p. 45)*.

N, B., & M, W. (2006 , Jun-Aug). *The effectiveness of a 15 minute weekly massage in reducing physical and psychological stress in nurses*. Retrieved June 29, 2014, from

PubMed.gov:
http://www.ncbi.nlm.nih.gov/pubmed/1680021
7

NHS. (2012). *Atlas of Variation for Healthcare.*
Retrieved June 29, 2014, from NHS Rightcare:
http://www.rightcare.nhs.uk/index.php/atlas/at
las-of-variation-2011/

Smith, T. W., Uchino, B. N., Berg, C. A.,
Florsheim, P., Pearce, G., Hawkins, M., et al.
(2009, June). *Conflict and collaboration in
middle-aged and older couples: II.
Cardiovascular reactivity during marital
interaction Vol 24(2), Jun 2009, 274-286.* .
Retrieved June 29, 2014, from American
Psychological Association:
http://psycnet.apa.org/journals/pag/24/2/274/

Stress in the Workplace. (2002). Retrieved June
28, 2014, from Royal Society for The Prevention
of Accidents:
http://www.rospa.com/occupationalsafety/advic
eandinformation/occupationalhealth/stress.aspx

*Stress-related and psychological disorders in
Great Britain (GB).* (n.d.). Retrieved June 28,
2014, from Health and Safety Executive:
http://www.hse.gov.uk/statistics/causdis/stress
/

The Numbers Count: Mental Disorders in America. (n.d.). Retrieved June 28, 2014, from National Institute of Mental Health: http://www.nimh.nih.gov/health/publications/the-numbers-count-mental-disorders-in-america/index.shtml

Walen Heather R, L. M. (2000). Social Support and Strain from Partner, Family, and Friends: Costs and Benefits for Men and Women in Adulthood. *Journal of Social and Personal Relationships.* , 17:5–30.

Woods, D. (2010, Nov 04). *Workers suffering from stress lie to their bosses when they feel unable to go to work.* Retrieved June 28, 2014, from HR Magazine: http://www.hrmagazine.co.uk/hro/news/1018662/workers-suffering-stress-lie-bosses-feel-unable

www.stress.org – American Institute of Stress.

Jill Bruce Diploma of Aromatherapy

The Garden of Eden.

www.ingramcontent.com/pod-product-compliance
Lightning Source LLC
Chambersburg PA
CBHW070917290526
45795CB00001B/340